CLINICAL LABORATORY SCIENCE IN THE CHANGING SCENE OF HEALTH CARE

CLINICAL LABORATORY SCIENCE IN THE CHANGING SCENE OF HEALTH CARE

Edited by JP Ashby
Department of Clinical Chemistry
Northwick Park Hospital and Clinical Research Centre
Harrow, Middlesex, UK

Proceedings of the sixth ECCLS Seminar held at Cologne, West Germany, 8th–10th May, 1985

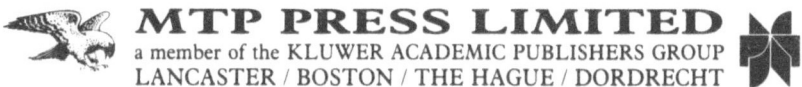

MTP PRESS LIMITED
a member of the KLUWER ACADEMIC PUBLISHERS GROUP
LANCASTER / BOSTON / THE HAGUE / DORDRECHT

Published in the UK and Europe by
MTP Press Limited
Falcon House
Lancaster, England

British Library Cataloguing in Publication Data

ECCLS Seminar   (6th : Cologne)
    Clinical laboratory science in the changing
    scene of health care : proceedings of the
    sixth ECCLS Seminar held at Cologne, West
    Germany, 1985.
    1. Diagnosis, Laboratory
    I. Title   II. Ashby, J.P.
    616.07'5   RB37

ISBN-13: 978-94-010-7934-1   e-ISBN-13: 978-94-009-3197-8
DOI:10.1007/978-94-009-3197-8

Published in the USA by
MTP Press
A division of Kluwer Academic Publishers
101 Philip Drive
Norwell, MA 02061, USA

Library of Congress Cataloging-in-Publication Data

ECCLS Seminar (6th : 1985 : Cologne, Germany)
    Clinical laboratory science in the changing scene
of health care.

    Includes bibliographies.
    1. Diagnosis, Laboratory--Philosphophy--Congresses.
2. Medical care--Congresses. I. Ashby, J.P.
II. European Committee for Clinical Laboratory Standards.
III. Title. [DNLM: 1. Delivery of Health Care--
trends--congresses. 2. Technology, Medical--trends--
congresses. W3 EC9 6th 1985c / QY 21 E17 1985c]
RB37.A2E29   1985   616.07'5   86-21150

Contents

CONTENTS

Preface

The sixth ECCLS seminar was held in May 1985 at Walberberg near Cologne. It was perhaps appropriate that almost six years after its inauguration, ECCLS should stand back and look at the changing scene in health care, examine its impact on clinical laboratory science and assess the requirements for further written and material standards in laboratory practice.

The seminar highlighted the increasing economic pressures which many laboratory directors now face, emphasizing the need for accurate and reliable management information. It became apparent that the extent to which standardization has been introduced into the different laboratory disciplines is variable and although a considerable amount has already been achieved, it is clear that much yet remains to be done: it is the definition of future requirements which constitutes the principal message of this book.

As with previous ECCLS seminars the speakers were chosen for their acknowledged expertise in their own fields. Editorial changes to the papers presented in this volume have been made only to ensure consistency in the style of presentation.

JP Ashby

List of Contributors

JE BARCLAY
Technicon International Div.
6-10 Quai de Seine
93200 St. Denis
France

I BATTY
Wellcome Research Laboratories
Langley Court
Beckenham
Kent
UK

AE BENNETT
Health and Safety Directorate
Commission of European
    Communities
Batiment Jean Monnet
Plateque du Kirchberg
BP 1907
Luxembourg

A BERLIN
Health and Safety Directorate
Commission of European
    Communities
Batiment Jean Monnet
Plateque du Kirchberg
BP 1907
Luxembourg

SS BROWN
West Midlands Regional
    Laboratory for Toxicology
Dudley Road Hospital
Birmingham
UK

DH CALAM
National Institute for Biological
    Standards and Control
Holly Hill
London
UK

M HJELM
Department of Clinical
    Biochemistry
Institute of Child Health
Guildford Street
London
UK

WJ HUNTER
Health and Safety Directorate
Commission of European
    Communities
Batiment Jean Monnet
Plateque du Kirchberg
BP 1907
Luxembourg

OAN HUSAIN
Regional Cytology Centre
St. Stephen's Hospital
Chelsea
London
UK

KS JOHANSEN
World Health Organization
Regional Office for Europe
8 Scherfigsvej
DK-2100 Copenhagen
Denmark

LIST OF CONTRIBUTORS

G KOKHOLM
Radiometer A/S
Copenhagen
Denmark

B LEIJNSE
Department of Chemical
    Pathology
Erasmus University
Rotterdam
The Netherlands

SM LEWIS
Department of Haematology
Royal Postgraduate Medical
    School
Du Cane Road
London
UK

JG LINES
William Harvey Hospital
Ashford
Kent
UK

RG NADEAU
EM Diagnostics Systems Inc
480 Democrat Road
Gibbstown, NJ 08027
USA

R NETTER
Laboratoire National de la
    Santé
25, boulevard Saint-Jacques
75680 Paris Cedex 14
France

M ROTH
Central Laboratory of Clinical
    Chemistry
Hôpital Cantonal Universitaire
CH-1211 Geneve 4
Switzerland

J RYGAARD
Patologisk-Anatomisk Institut
Kommunehospitalet
DK-1399 Copenhagen K
Denmark

N SANDERS
William Harvey Hospital
Ashford
Kent
UK

AHW WAHBA
World Health Organization
Regional Office for Europe
8 Scherfigsvej
DK-2100 Copenhagen
Denmark

JGW WITTKÄMPER
Institut für
    Politikwissenschaft
der Westfalischen Wilhelms-
    Universität
D-4400 Münster
FRG

Part 1

CURRENT CONCEPTS OF HEALTH AND HEALTH CARE

1

A European Overview of the Health Care Scene

KS Johansen

THE PRESENT SITUATION

General socioeconomic developments and - perhaps to a somewhat lesser degree - improved health care, have led to an improvement in key health issues. Life expectancy at birth is between 65 and 73 years for men and 72 and 80 years for women. However, in the less developed, southern areas of Europe, the life expectancy is lower - around 52 years for men and 55 years for women.

Although differences exist between the countries and areas of Europe, it is becoming more and more apparent that a rapid social change, coupled with a high standard of living and accelerating technological developments, leads to fundamental lifestyle and environmental changes, with resulting serious health implications. The rapidly expanding car industry affects urban design, increases noise and chemical pollution of the environment, produces accidents characterized by a high death rate and severe disabilities, and reduces drastically the physical activities of daily life. Of major importance in Europe, also, is the high prevalence of cigarette smoking, which is clearly associated with several types of cancer and with cardiovascular diseases. Another matter of great concern is the abuse of alcohol, which is an important cause of road and work accidents; it is also associated with mental illness and suicide and plays an aggravating role in several major diseases. The abuse of other drugs constitutes a serious and growing problem in most countries. Obesity and unbalanced nutrition are major problems in the more affluent countries of Europe, while the lack of nutrients leads to stunted growth in the poorer countries. A high incidence of sexually transmitted diseases has accompanied changing lifestyles and sexual attitudes. Lack of physical exercise, a frequent result of more affluent lifestyles, may well prove to be an important factor in ill-health. The rapid introduction of new chemicals in increasing quantities, which affect air, water, food and the working environment, has posed new problems of risk identification, surveillance and control. The wider use of nuclear energy involves potential risks from radiation

3

hazards.

The instability of the family creates insecure conditions for children and leaves many people isolated or lonely. The rapidly growing trend for women to take up work outside the home has altered the role of the family in providing care for children, the aged and the disabled. Individuals become more exposed and vulnerable as moral and behavioural rules change and social and economic barriers diminish. Social tensions arise from the presence of underprivileged immigrant groups, especially if their norms and ways of living differ from those of the rest of the population. A relative poverty of some members of the community and rapidly increasing unemployment, especially in the younger age groups, has also shown adverse effects on health.

In nearly all European countries the services are biased towards secondary and tertiary levels of health care at the expense of the primary level. High-technology hospitals tend to be concentrated in the main cities. Moreover, health care in hospitals is often criticized for being dehumanizing, impersonal and overtechnical.

Insufficiently assessed technological development may result in an increase in iatrogenic problems, including malpractice, hospital infection, and accidents due to excessive or inappropriate use of drugs. It may also lead to an increase in the professional monopoly of health knowledge and a reduction in self-reliance. Social security payment systems and the sales promotion practices of some manufacturers may also encourage the excessive use of diagnostic tests, equipment, pharmaceuticals and other forms of medical intervention.

Last but not least, community participation is virtually non-existent in the primary health care systems of most European countries, with a resulting fragmented system of health care without a pattern of referral.

Entitlement under social security schemes and health service systems has been steadily increasing throughout Europe, but only in a minority of countries does coverage extend to 100% of the population. Where social security systems exclude the more affluent section of the population, private health insurance generally fills that gap, sometimes to the detriment of the social service system of health care, as personnel may be attracted to more remunerative private practices.

In many European countries there is still a lack of clear health policies, a limited structure for health planning, and an insufficient system for evaluating development plans or their implementation. There is, moreover, little cooperation with other socioeconomic sectors.

FUTURE TRENDS

There is no doubt that the present situation in health care needs more concentrated efforts by the various partners in health care, namely patients and community, health authorities, professions, third party providers, industry and the media. Information and communication channels must be improved, research and develop-

4

ment ought to be guided towards real needs, budgets based on rationality, quality and population coverage and utilization of services properly monitored.

European countries will have to continue to adjust to the altered competitive position of their economics and to further major changes in production processes, which are likely to be significant features of the next two decades. There is also likely to be more geographical movement of the population in search of employment opportunities, making communities still more unstable.

A GLOBAL STRATEGY

The recent creation of the global programme for appropriate health care technology meshes into WHO's worldwide Health For All strategy and its targets. These propose that by the late eighties each Member State should have worked out its technology assessment needs, and by the late nineties it should have access to an operational mechanism for systematic monitoring and evaluation. These general principles will be underpinned by a new awareness of how clinical practice, health management and budgeting exercises can all draw on the benefits of overall evaluation.

Proper involvement of all parts of the community will help to assess the appropriateness of the technology. Appropriate health care technology is a major area in which technical cooperation and transfer amongst countries is vital.

The programme operates through a network of institutions and resource people involved in common projects dealing with specific problems. Its aims are to identify technologies in need of assessment, whether already in use, or under development or forecast; to develop methods for assessing technology by studies and literature review; to convene consensus groups; to analyse, validate and disseminate information; to publish reports with global implications; to establish contacts with governments, intergovernmental and nongovernmental organizations, industry and consumer groups; to develop national models to advise on standards for quality assurance; to promote educational efforts aimed at providing health workers, policy makers and the public with a proper understanding of health care technology and the problems of its transfer, and to promote contacts with the mass media as well as specialized journals, media and industry.

In collaboration with member countries, industry, insurance companies, health professionals and consumer groups, the following key issues have been identified as those with high priority:

(1)   Communication technologies: information and computers in health care, health policy and management;

(2)   Comparative variation in health care practice;

(3)   Budgetary incentives and disincentives for appropriate use of technologies;

(4)   Assessment and use of medical technologies: methodology and insulin pumps;

(5)   Laboratory technologies;

(6)   Imaging technologies: basic radiological system (BRS) and

magnetic resonance imaging (MRI);
(7)   Perinatal technologies;
(8)   Safety in health care: hospital infection control, biosafety and prevention of allergy;
(9)   Drug utilization: antibiotics, iron.

2

Is there a European Concept of Health and Health Care?

JGW Wittkämper

INTRODUCTION

A European concept may be one of an international non-governmental organization (INGO) or one of an international governmental organization (IGO). There are innumerable sets of INGO documents concerning health and health care, e.g. of church organizations or of trade unions.

This paper deals with the IGO concepts available in Europe for which there are two main sources. One source is in Strasbourg, at the Council of Europe with its 21 member states. This, the oldest institution of European integration, has a special department for health and health care whose recommendations comprise more than 3000 pages. The second source is in Brussels, at the EEC, with only limited and in most cases implied powers in the fields of health and health care. Nevertheless, there are clear-cut fields of EEC activity concerning health and health care, with which this paper will deal.

THE COUNCIL OF EUROPE

Established by ten nations on 5th May 1949 as Europe's first political institution, with the first international parliamentary forum in history, the Council of Europe today has twenty-one member states: Austria, Belgium, Cyprus, Denmark, France, the Federal Republic of Germany, Greece, Iceland, Ireland, Italy, Liechtenstein, Luxembourg, Malta, the Netherlands, Norway, Portugal, Spain, Sweden, Switzerland, Turkey and the United Kingdom.
   The Council of Europe's aim is to achieve a greater unity between its members for the purposes of safeguarding and realizing the ideals and principles which are their common heritage, and of facilitating their economic and social progress. The pursuit of that objective is the responsibility of two bodies - the Committee of Ministers and the Consultative Assembly - assisted by a corps of

technical and administrative services, viz. the secretariat.

The scope of the Council of Europe's competence under its statute is vast, since only defence questions are excluded. Its activities touch on every aspect of life in Europe and find expression in many forms, such as recommendations and resolutions addressed to, and conventions and agreements concluded between all member states. Where, however, a lesser number of states wish to engage in some action in which not all their European partners desire to join, they can conclude a partial agreement which is binding on themselves alone.

It was on this basis that the partial agreement in the social and public health fields was concluded under Resolution (59) 23, adopted on 16th November 1959 by the Council of Europe Committee of Ministers. The following states acceded to the partial agreement: Belgium, France, the Federal Republic of Germany, Italy, Luxembourg, the Netherlands and the United Kingdom. They have continued, within the Council of Europe, the social work hitherto undertaken by the Brussels Treaty Organization and then by Western European Union. Austria, Denmark, Ireland and Switzerland acceded to the partial agreement activities in the public health field, and Greece, Norway and Sweden to certain of them. Spain has acceded to the administrative arrangements for the health control of sea, air and land traffic and to the European agreement on the restriction of the use of certain detergents in washing and cleaning products. Austria participates in the social and rehabilitation activities of the partial agreement. Norway, Portugal, Spain and Switzerland participate in the rehabilitation activities.

The activities in the three main areas dealing with the protection of public health, the rehabilitation and resettlement of disabled people and the promotion of intergovernmental cooperation in the social field are entrusted to committees of experts who are in turn responsible to steering committees for each of the three areas.

Protection of public health

In the field of public health, the Council of Europe works in five fields.

(1) Food and food hygiene, comprising food additives, intentional additives, unintentional additives, food packaging components, residues from pesticides, residues from drugs, environmental or accidental contaminants, and food hygiene.

(2) Cosmetic products and their ingredients.

(3) Pesticides, including pesticide registration, and safe handling and use of pesticides.

(4) Pharmaceutical questions, including patient information and consumer health, European pharmacopoeia, clinical pharmacology, and general work such as terms and classifications.

(5)   Medical questions, including epidemiology of communicable diseases, health control of sea, air and land traffic, congenital anomalies, and cancer.

(From document P-SG (85) 5)

The Conference of European Ministers of Health

At the Conference of European Ministers responsible for health (Madrid, September 1981), the Spanish Minister of Labour, Health and Social Security, stressed the need to lay down practical principles for a European approach to health in his opening address as follows:

> The work carried out during the last thirty years under the auspices of the World Health Organization's Regional Office for Europe and of the Council of Europe means that we can also count on technical support in achieving that fuller co-operation which will allow us to consider laying down a number of standards for the purpose of giving practical effect to this European approach to the promotion of health.
>   I have examined the set of resolutions and recommendations which the Council of Europe has circulated to us and I see that much of the groundwork for such standards has already been done, as far as structures, institutions, staff and finance are concerned. This applies not only to the various branches of curative medicine, but also to prevention in its primary, secondary and tertiary forms, as well as their social implications.
>   I feel that this standard-setting work might culminate in a text which we, as Ministers of Health, might adopt at one of our future conferences and which might then serve as a kind of guideline for a European health policy. This policy would lie somewhere between the purely national approach and the worldwide approach embodied in WHO's campaign for 'health for all by the year 2000' ....

At the same opening session, Mr G Adinolfi, Deputy Secretary General of the Council of Europe, welcomed the initiative taken by the Spanish Minister of Labour, Health and Social Security and added that:

> unanimous acceptance of these principles is bound to facilitate codification of current international standards and practice in the matter of the protection, promotion and improvement of health, having regard in particular to the texts adopted by the Committees of Ministers and the World Health Organization and without losing sight of the differences in levels of development which exist between our member states. This will also mean

9

that a constant watch will have to be kept on the effectiveness of these standards and on their utility with a view to the convergence of national health programmes in Europe.

At the end of their conference, the European ministers responsible for public health adopted conclusions on a number of points which might provide a basis for a European strategy for the prevention of sickness and promotion of health in the years ahead. It recommended, inter alia, that the Committee of Ministers of the Council of Europe should draw up 'European guidelines for the promotion of health, including standards'. The Committee of Ministers decided in December 1981 to send to the European Health Committee (CDSP) the recommendations made to it by the conference concerning activities to be undertaken in the years ahead, which the CDSP then accepted.

It should also be noted that Objective 15.1 in the second medium-term-plan (1981-1986) calls for the preparation of an European health promotion programme in the following terms:

Such a programme will require:

- The codification of existing international standards and practices in the protection, promotion and improvement of health, with special reference to texts adopted by the Committee of Ministers and the World Health Organization, taking into account the different levels of development of member states.

- The continuous monitoring of the effectiveness of these standards and their relevance to the convergence of national health care programmes in Europe.

- On the basis of the above-mentioned considerations, the development of principles in areas of health policy.

On the CDSP's proposal, approved by the Committee of Ministers, an activity was included in the Programme of Intergovernmental Activities from 1983 onwards (Document MSN 2-6).

The CDSP's major activities over the last 25 years (MSN 2-6)

The main areas of activity over the past 25 years have been:

(1) Principles concerning planning (coordination and integration), management and assessment:

    (a) Planning levels and role of each level;
    (b) Specific aspects: balance between care in and outside hospitals.

(2) Primary health care - training and roles:

    (a) The basic health care team and its role;

    (b)   The general practitioner;
    (c)   The nurse;
    (d)   The social worker;
    (e)   Other supporting staff in primary health care i.e. the psychologist, care in the family, and self-care.

(3)   Other health care staff categories:

    (a)   The specialist doctor;
    (b)   Medical laboratory technicians.

(4)   Hospital services

    (a)   Planning: different types of hospitals and hospital groups;
    (b)   The international structure and management of hospitals.

(5)   Preventive and other services (mainly in somatic medicine) for special purposes or for special groups (including out-patient hospital services):

    (a)   Family planning;
    (b)   Perinatal surveillance;
    (c)   Child health surveillance;
    (d)   Accidents in childhood;
    (e)   School health services;
    (f)   Dental health;
    (g)   Sexually transmitted diseases;
    (h)   Preventive screening for adults.

(6)   Protection and promotion of mental health:

    (a)   Organization of preventive services in mental illness (including care);
    (b)   Prevention of alcohol-related problems (with some reference to smoking);
    (c)   Prevention of drug-related problems.

An example of European cooperation in the field of blood

The Committee of Experts on Blood Transfusion and Immuno-haematology was created in 1962, although the first seeds of European cooperation in the blood transfusion field were sown as long ago as 1953. The work is carried out in close and fruitful collaboration with the WHO, the League of Red Cross Societies, the Order of Malta and the International Society for Blood Transfusion. In order to pursue objectives as effectively as possible in these highly technical fields, the committee has made use of three subordinate bodies which are responsible respectively for:

-    following developments in the automation, computerization and quality control in blood transfusion services;

- drawing up standards for the European reference reagents used to define histocompatability;

- studying current problems in the fields of blood transfusion and immunohaematology by means of a team of experts visiting the main centres in Europe.

In addition, European courses in blood transfusion techniques and on aspects of histocompatibility testing have been set up to meet training needs.   The European Histocompatibility Training Conference met in Strasbourg for the first time in 1983.

The European agreements on blood problems aim at standardizing and facilitating the rapid exchange of blood and blood products on a non-profit basis:

(1)   European Agreement 26 on the Exchange of Therapeutic Substances of Human Origin was ready for signature in 1958 and is at present in force in 17 of the Council of Europe member states.   Its aim is the standardization of therapeutic substances of human origin, the abolition of customs duties on non-commercial blood supplies and the uniform labelling of all supplies sent from one country to another.   A protocol to the agreement, which is regularly revised by the Committee of Experts on Blood Transfusion and Immunohaematology, describes the minimum requirements each substance should meet.

(2)   European Agreement 39 on the Exchange of Blood Grouping Reagents provides for the availability, on a non-commercial basis, of such reagents whenever the need may arise. Opened for signature in 1962, this agreement is now in force in 16 Council of Europe member states.   Minimum requirements blood grouping reagents should meet are described in a protocol to the agreement.   The committee of experts is at present reviewing the protocol section dealing with human anti-globulin reagents.

(3)   A third European Agreement (84), opened for signature in September 1974, is designed to facilitate the exchange of sera for the determination of histocompatibility.   It has been ratified by eight member states and signed by four.   A list of national and regional tissue-typing reference laboratories in member states and Finland is issued annually by the Council of Europe.   These laboratories use the same research techniques and reagents from the same sources to determine blood and tissue (HLA) groups.

An initial panel of reference tissue-typing reagents has been set up to establish acceptable methods of selection.   The aim of such a European panel is to define the specificity of tissue-typing reagents.   This European agreement and its protocol facilitate and legalize the exchange of standardized reagents on a European level and establish the minimum requirements.   It will eventually lead to the formation, on a

European scale, of large pools of patients who are potential recipients of one or more organs.

Measures recommended
by the Committee of Experts on
Blood Transfusion and Immunohaematology

(1) Recommendation on instruction in blood transfusion (1963 and 1964)

(2) Recommended measures on active immunization (1964)

(3) Recommended measures on the standardization of blood grouping sera (1965)

(4) Recommended measures on Australia Antigen (1971)

(5) Recommended measures on minimal requirements for blood donors (1972 and 1973)

(6) Recommended measures on expressing results of antibody quantitation (1973)

(7) Recommended measures on the quality control of sera used as tissue-typing reagents (1973, 1974 and 1976)

(8) Recommended measures on antigen variants of the Rh system (1973)

(9) Recommended measures on prevention of maternal Rh-immunization and sensitisation (1973 and 1976)

(10) Recommended measures on the organization of blood transfusion (1973)

(11) Recommended measures on the introduction of inert plastics (1974)

(12) Recommended measures on the declaration of the origin of raw materials used in the preparation of plasma fractions (1975)

(13) Guidelines for the organization of blood transfusion services (1975)

(14) Recommendations on the quantitative determination of erythrocytic antibodies (1976)

(15) Recommendation on the quality of Fresh Frozen Plasma used for the treatment of acute bleeding disorders (1981)

(16) Recommendation on the use of Fluosol-Da (1981).

CLINICAL LABORATORY SCIENCE IN HEALTH CARE

THE EEC

Health politics do not represent an explicit area of the EEC. Nevertheless, there are four competences of the EEC in this field:

(1) Under Article 235 of the treaty, the EEC has implied powers in all fields where health questions are implied in an explicit area of competence.

(2) Under Articles 117 ss, the EEC holds vast powers in the fields of social security, and systems of social security and public health.

(3) Its competences in the field of science and technology, currently in the 1984-1987 programme, include the area of science and research in the fields of health and medicine, comprising four concerted actions which include the improvement of living and working conditions and the protection of health at the working place.

(4) A fourth area of EEC activity is the integration of professional law and standards concerning the 600,000 medical doctors, 800,000 nurses, 107,000 dentists, and 50,000 midwives in the EEC.

The EEC has taken both legal and administrative action in four areas covering pharmaceutical products, dangerous substances, cosmetic products and the health protection of working people. There is a lot of current work covering other areas.

The basis of the EEC activity was created in CD 75/365, which states:

A committee of senior officials on public health, hereinafter called the 'committee', shall be set up within the Commission. The committee shall consist of senior officials from the member states who have direct responsibility in the field of public health. The tasks of the committee shall be:

- To collect all relevant information on the conditions under which general and specialist medical care is given in the member states;

- To deliver opinions which could guide the Commission's work with a view to amendment of the above mentioned directives.

In 1981 (C287/32) the European Parliament recommended that a health card should be introduced, as a first practical step, for individuals who are particularly at risk i.e. persons who are suffering from serious and chronic diseases and who for that reason stand in special need of swift and appropriate medical attention. The introduction of a health card at European level would provide valuable experience, in particular with regard to the willingness of the European medical profession to help to ensure that such cards

14

are always kept up to date.

Pharmaceutical products

The Commission of the European Communities set up a number of rules governing medicaments in the European Community. The primary purpose of the Community rules relating to medicinal products is to safeguard public health whilst at the same time ensuring that the development of the pharmaceutical industry and trade in medicinal products will not be hindered.

(1) Council Directives 65/65/EEC, 75/318/ EEC and 75/319 EEC lay down common rules governing the most important aspects of the marketing of proprietary medicinal products for human use in the ten member states, including:

    (a) Conditions for marketing authorizations: requirements for tests and trials to be carried out on proprietary medicinal products for human use;

    (b) Manufacture and control of proprietary medicinal products for human use;

    (c) Labelling and package leaflets;

    (d) Supervisory duties of national authorities;

    (e) The creation of the Committee for Proprietary Medicinal Products to ensure cooperation between the competent national authorities with a view to obviating inconsistent national decisions relating to marketing authorizations which are still issued at national level.

(2) Council Directive 83/570/EEC makes some important modifications to these rules, including:

    (a) The introduction of evaluation reports and data sheets;

    (b) The introduction of tests for bioavailability and mutagenicity;

    (c) Major changes in the procedure of the Committee for Proprietary Medicinal Products after November 1985.

(3) Council Recommendation 83/571/EEC contains notes for guidance on the conduct of certain tests and trials for proprietary medicinal products for human use. Further notes for guidance are at an advanced stage of preparation and will be published in due course.

(4) Council Directive 78/25/EEC, as amended, specifies the colouring matters which may be used in medicinal products for both human and veterinary use.

(5)   To advise the Commission on general questions in the field of proprietary medicinal products, Council Decision 75/320/EEC created the Pharmaceutical Committee consisting of senior national public health officials.

(6)   In addition to these basic legislative texts other documents of general interest relating to proprietary medicinal products for human use are:

(a)   the Commission communication on parallel imports of proprietary medicinal products for which marketing authorizations have already been granted;

(b)   the notice to applicants for marketing authorizations for proprietary medicinal products explaining how to use the current C.P.M.P. procedure.

(7)   Council Directives 81/851/EEC and 81/852/EEC, which came into force in October 1983, lay down the rules relating to veterinary medicinal products. Based on the rules applying to human medicines, they include:

(a)   Conditions for marketing authorizations and requirements for tests and trials to be carried out on veterinary medicines;

(b)   Labelling and package leaflets;

(c)   Supervisory duties of national authorities;

(d)   The creation of the Committee for Veterinary Medicinal Products to ensure cooperation between the competent national authorities with a view to obviating inconsistent national decisions relating to marketing authorizations which are still issued at national level.

Nevertheless there are differences between the human and veterinary sectors caused, in particular, by the need to avoid the presence of harmful residues from veterinary medicines in food intended for human consumption.

Dangerous substances

The main activities in this field were the Council Directives:

(1)   of 27th June 1967 on the approximation of laws, regulations and administrative provisions relating to the classification, packing and labelling of dangerous substances (67/548/EEC);

(2)   of 21st December 1978 prohibiting the placing on the market and the use of plant protection products containing certain active substances (79/117/EEC);

(3)   of 27th July 1976 on the approximation of the laws, regulations and administrative provisions of the member states relating to restrictions on the marketing and use of certain dangerous substances and preparations (76/769/EEC).

Cosmetic products

The activity in this field is on the approximation of the laws.

Health protection of working people

The main activities in this field are the following Council Directives:

(1)   of 1st June 1976 laying down the revised basic safety standards for the health protection of the general public and workers against the dangers of ionizing radiation (76/579/Euratom) with many amendments e.g. 80/836;

(2)   of 29th June 1978 on an action programme of the European Communities on safety and health at work. The main aim of the programme is to increase the level of protection against occupational risks of all types by increasing the efficiency of measures for preventing, monitoring and controlling these risks. Such a programme should make it possible to achieve the following general objectives:

   (a)   Improvement of the working situation with a view to increased safety and with due regard to health requirements in the organization of the work. Such an improvement should cover not only the existing situation but also new technical developments. In order to monitor more effectively the application of preventive measures, surveillance of health and working conditions must be intensified, notably in line with the exigencies of occupational medicine, hygiene and safety appropriate to present-day conditions;

   (b)   Improvement of knowledge in order to identify and assess risks and perfect prevention and control methods;

   (c)   Improvement of human attitudes in order to promote and develop safety and health consciousness.

(3)   of 18th March 1980 adopting a research and training programme (1980-1984) for the European Atomic Energy Community in the field of biology health protection (Radiation Protection Programme) (80/342/Euratom);

(4)   of 19th December 1978 on the approximation of the laws of the member states relating to the determination of the noise

of construction plant and equipment (79/113/EEC).

Other current activities

These cover the following problems:

(1)   A proposal for a council directive laying down basic measures for the radiation protection of persons undergoing medical examinations or treatment (submitted by the Commission to the Council on 18th December 1980);

(2)   A proposal for a second council directive on the protection of workers from the risks related to exposure to agents at work, an example being asbestos (submitted by the Commission to the Council on 26th September 1980);

(3)   A proposal for a council directive laying down basic standards for the health protection of workers and the general public against the dangers of microwave radiation (submitted by the Commission to the Council on 26th June 1980);

(4)   A council directive of 27th November 1980 on the protection of workers from the risks related to exposure to chemical, physical and biological agents at work (80/1107/EEC);

(5)   A council directive of 28th July 1982 on the protection of workers from the risks related to exposure to metallic lead and its ionic compounds at work (first individual directive within the meaning of Article 8 of Directive 80/1107/EEC) (82/605/EEC);

(6)   A council directive of 28th September 1981 on the approximation of the laws of the member states relating to analytical, pharmaco-toxicological and clinical standards and protocols in respect of the testing of veterinary medicinal products (81/852/EEC).

CONCLUSIONS

As far as the EEC is concerned, we have only the beginning of the beginning of a European health policy, but the Council of Europe - despite holding no executive competence - has done much to shape a European health policy, and we are near to completing a framework for such a policy on the Council of Europe level.

3

The Effects of Health and Safety Legislation on the Practice of Clinical Laboratory Science

A Berlin, AE Bennett and WJ Hunter

INTRODUCTION

For more than a decade there has been considerable interest at European Community level in the quantitative assessment of biological indicators in relation to environmental, occupational and public health.

This interest and concern has developed at different levels:

- Assessment of the health significance of the biological parameters both in qualitative and quantitative terms;

- Development of methods and reference materials;

- Establishment of quality assurance programmes.

Abbreviations used in the text

ALA	Delta-aminolaevulinic acid	IUPAC	International Union of Pure and Applied Chemistry
ALAD	Delta-aminolaevulinic acid dehydratase		
		NIOSH	National Institute of Occupational Safety and Health
ALAU	Delta-aminolaevulinic acid in urine		
CEC	Commission of European Communities	OSHA	Occupational Safety and Health Agency
ILO	International Labour Organization	UNEP	United Nations Environmental Programme
IPCS	International Programme on Chemical Safety	ZPP	Zinc protoporphyrin

---

In 1975 at the International Conference of Environmental Sensing and Assessment, a review of the various quality control and harmonization programmes at European Community level was presented[1]. This review included nine programmes devoted to biological tissues ranging from heavy metals in blood and urine, to organochlorine pesticides in fatty materials, carboxyhaemoglobin determinations and ALA in urine.

ENVIRONMENTAL HEALTH

In 1977 an international workshop on the use of biological specimens for the assessment of human exposure to environmental pollutants was held in Luxembourg, organized jointly by the Commission of the European Communities, the World Health Organization and the United States Environmental Protection Agency[2]. Using a broad interpretation of biological monitoring the workshop provided a summary (Table 3.1) of pollutants and human biological tissues amenable at present to biological monitoring.

Table 3.1 Pollutants and human biological tissues amenable at present to biological monitoring

Tissues \ Pollutants	Arsenic	Cadmium	Chromium	Lead	Inorganic Mercury	Methyl Mercury	Carbon Monoxide	Organochlorine Pesticides	Pentachlorophenol	Polychlorinated biphenyls	Chlorinated solvents	Benzene
Adipose tissue								x		x		
Blood	x	x		x	x	x	x	x		x	x	x
Bone				x								
Brain					x	x						
Expired air							x				x	x
Faeces		x										
Hair	x			x		x						
Kidney		x		x	x							
Liver		x		x		x						
Milk								x		x		
Placenta		x		x								
Teeth				x								
Urine	x	x	x	x	x				x		x	x

Simultaneously a directive on the 'Biological Screening of the Population for Lead', to be considered not only as a pilot programme in the field of biological monitoring but also a means of protecting the populations most exposed to lead was adopted by the Council of Ministers in March 1977[3]. The directive specifies that this screening shall be performed through the measurement of lead or ALAD in blood, and the results of the analyses are to be assessed in terms of the reference levels in Table 3.2.

THE EFFECTS OF HEALTH AND SAFETY LEGISLATION

Table 3.2 Reference levels for analyses of blood lead or ALAD

Reference levels	Median	90th Percentile	98th Percentile
PbB (μg/100 mL)	20	30	35
ALAD (EU)	35	25	20

The directive further stipulates that:

- The sampling is to be carried out on volunteers;

- There shall be groups of at least 100 persons examined in urban areas of more than 500,000 inhabitants;

- Groups of at least 100 persons shall be chosen where feasible from among people exposed to significant pollution;

- Other critical groups shall be examined as determined by the member states;

- In each member state, and during each campaign, the number of analyses to be performed shall be 50 or more per million inhabitants.

To ensure accuracy and comparability of results a continuous quality control programme was established in 1978 for the blood lead measurements, and a European standard method developed for the determination of delta-aminolaevulinic acid dehydratase[4].

If the reference levels are exceeded the directive requires member states to:

- Check the validity of the results;

- Take action to trace the exposure sources responsible for the levels being exceeded (this shall also include special attention devoted to all individuals with a blood lead level over 35 μg per 100 mL);

- Take all appropriate measures at the discretion of the competent national authorities.

The overall results are summarized in Table 3.3 and data for selected cities are given in Table 3.4[5].

Table 3.3 Overall results of CEC biological screening of the population for lead

Total number of subjects	Median lead level (μg/dL)	Number of subjects with PbB of 30 μg/dL	Number of subjects with PbB of 35/μg/dL
17,609	13	367 (2%)	184 (1%)

The main conclusions of the survey are:

- In general blood lead levels for the population examined in the European Community were lower than could have been anticipated from earlier fragmentary studies;

- The studies conducted in urban areas with no known specific source of lead (point emission sources from industry, plumbosolvency and lead pipes) seem to indicate that there is no serious risk for the population, taking into account the reference values provided for in the directive;

- Studies conducted in areas with known specific sources, and in particular for critical population groups such as children of lead workers or children living near lead works, have confirmed that a health risk may exist since in some of those instances reference levels have been exceeded. This has been the case for known problem areas and for newly-found potential problem areas. Member states are taking active measures to circumscribe the problem areas and are taking remedial action where necessary.

OCCUPATIONAL HEALTH

With the increasing use of clinical and biological parameters in occupational health practice, a growing concern has developed among the workforce and the trade unions with the routine monitoring of certain biological parameters. While recognizing that biological monitoring can contribute to a better assessment of an individual worker's exposure to a given chemical agent, trade unions seem to be in general concerned with the misuse which can be made of the results. To ensure the best practical use of such monitoring there is a need strictly to define the terminology, the scope and the use which can be made of the individual results.

Table 3.4 Blood lead (μg dL^{-1}) in non-exposed adults in selected cities

Zone	Nb	Men percentile 50	90	Nb Woman percentile 50	90
Belgium					
Brussel urban	75	19.0	25.0	47	16.0	21.0
Denmark					
Copenhagen	35	11.8	18.0	36	8.9	13.0
France					
Bordeaux	22	15.0	28.0	39	12.0	23.0
Lille	38	12.0	26.0	60	11.0	21.0
Lyon	96	15.0	24.0	110	11.0	19.0
Marseille	165	16.0	27.0	104	10.0	16.0
Nantes	20	15.5	25.5	69	9.0	20.0
Nice	40	14.0	24.0	57	10.0	15.0
Paris	350	17.0	27.0	424	12.0	19.0
Toulouse	51	13.0	21.0	54	10.0	16.0
Ireland					
Dublin	25	16.0	20.0	25	12.5	19.9
Italy					
Bologna	68	21.0	35.0	32	11.0	20.8
Milan	122	18.0	28.0	277	13.0	19.0
Naples	98	21.0	28.0	100	15.0	20.8
Rome	241	20.0	28.0	180	15.0	21.9
Torino	84	20.0	38.0	112	15.0	23.0
Luxembourg					
Luxemburg	59	15.0	21.0	52	11.45	16.0
Netherlands					
Amsterdam	50	15.0	28.0	50	10.0	13.0
United Kingdom					
Inner B'ham	46	17.0	23.4	51	12.0	18.0
(Sparkbrook)					
Inner B'ham	55	16.0	24.5	44	11.5	18.6
(Handsworth)					
Leeds	55	17.0	26.0	45	13.0	21.0
Liverpool	43	15.0	25.0	57	12.0	20.0
London-Islington	39	14.0	20.1	48	10.0	14.4
London-Lambeth	95	15.0	20.0	105	10.0	15.0
Manchester	46	19.0	27.4	54	15.0	21.6
Sheffield	52	16.0	23.0	48	12.0	17.2
Federal Rep. Germany					
Hannover*	60	12.5	17.9	42	9.0	12.9
	44	10.0	15.9	39	8.0	12.0
Hamburg*	43	12.0	20.9	42	11.0	18.8
	22	12.0	18.9	42	11.5	16.9

Blood lead (μg dL^{-1}) in non-exposed adults in selected cities
* Inner urban areas with more than 500,000 inhabitants, from CEC (1981)

Following the 1977 seminar, in 1980 the Commission organized jointly with OSHA and NIOSH a seminar in Luxembourg on the roles of ambient and biological monitoring in the assessment of toxic agents at the workplace[6],[7]. At that seminar considerable attention was devoted to the definition of terms. The terms 'monitoring', 'ambient monitoring', 'biological monitoring' and 'health surveillance' were defined and these definitions serve at present as references at European Community level.

Monitoring is a systematic continuous or repetitive health-related activity designed to lead if necessary to corrective actions. Three types of monitoring are defined: ambient, biological and health surveillance.

Ambient monitoring is the measurement and assessment of agents at the workplace and evaluates ambient exposure and health risk compared to an appropriate reference.

Biological monitoring is the measurement and assessment of workplace agents or their metabolites either in tissues, secreta, excreta, expired air or any combination of these to evaluate exposure and health risk compared to an appropriate reference.

Health surveillance is the periodic medico-physiological examination of exposed workers with the objective of protecting health and preventing occupationally related disease. The detection of established disease is outside the scope of this definition.

The definitions of biological monitoring and health surveillance separate components of a continuum which can range from the measurement of agents in the body through measurements of metabolites, to signs of early disease.

In its programme on internationally recommended health-based limits in occupational exposure, WHO clearly recognized the importance of biological limits and the need to follow the above definitions closely. For the first three series of compounds - heavy metals[8], selected organic solvents[9] and pesticides[10] - nine biological limits were set. The biological indicators and limits recommended are summarized together with the ambient limits in Table 3.5.

To date only one community directive on occupational health has been adopted which includes biological lead monitoring[11],[12]. In addition to limiting the values for lead in air at work, the directive sets both action levels and limit values for blood lead and other associated indicators. A comparison of the biological levels proposed and adopted is presented in Table 3.6 and the provisions to be taken at various levels are set out in Table 3.7.

While the primary biological indicator is blood lead, there are supplementary indicators such as ALAD, ZPP and ALAU. For ALAU, the reference method selected was that of Davis and Andelman[13], taking into account the results of an intercomparison programme using different methods[14] (Table 3.8) and the further standardization of the Davis technique.

A questionnaire is now being finalized to seek information

Table 3.5 WHO-recommended health-based limits in occupational exposure

Category	Substance or compound	Ambient	Biological
Heavy metals	Cadmium	250 μg/m^3 (short term) 10 μg/m^3	5 μg Cd/g creatinine (urine) 5 μg Cd/L whole blood
	Inorganic lead	30-60 μg/m^3	400 μgPb/L whole blood 300 μgPb/L whole blood (females reproductive age)
	Manganese	0.3 mg/m^3	-
	Inorganic mercury	500 μg/m^3 (short term metallic mercury) 25 μg/m^3 (long term metallic mercury) 50 μg/m^3 (long term inorganic mercury)	50 μg/g creatinine
Selected organic solvents	Toluene	600-800 mg/m^3 (short term) 200-375 mg/cm^3 (long term)	1.5-2.5 ç of hippuric acid/g creatinine (urine)
	Xylene	215 mg/m^3 (long term)	1.4 g methylhippuric acid/L (urine)
	Carbon disulphide	60 mg/m^3 (short term) 10 mg/m^3 (long term) 3 mg/m^3 (long term- females fertile age)	-
	Trichlor-ethylene	1000 mg/m^3 (short term) 135 mg/m^3 (long term)	-
Pesticides	Nalathion	-	30% reduction in ChE activity (blood)
	Carbaryl Dinitro-o-cresol	0.3 mg/m^3 (long term)	0.02 mg lindane/L blood 20 mg DNOC/L blood

from all industries in the European Community involved with the handling of cadmium, regarding their current practices. In terms of industrial hygiene, special emphasis will be placed on the use of biological indicators.

Finally, to promote further the use of biological indicators at work for the protection of the workers' health, the Commission initiated in 1983 the publication of a series dealing with the assessment of human exposure to industrial chemicals. Two series have been published to date and a third is in preparation[15,16] (Table 3.9).

While we have been very restrictive in our definition of

Table 3.6 Proposed and adopted action levels and limit values for lead at work (Biological)

	Proposed	Adopted
Action levels	PbB 35 μg/100 mL (beyond this value the directive applies)	PbB 40 μg/100 mL (information)
		PbB 50 μg/100 mL (beyond this value full application of directive)
Limit values	PbB 35 μg/100 mL (pregnant workers at entry into force of directive)	PbB 70 μg/100 mL for PbB 70-80 μg/100 mL additional biological indicators
	PbB 45 μg/100 mL or	ALAU <20 mg/g
	ALAU 6 mg/L (potential pregnancy at entry into force of directive)	(creatinine)
		or ZPP < 20 mg/g
	PbB 70 μg/100 mL or	or ALAD > 6 EU (in 1986)
	ALAU 15 mg/L (at entry into force of directive) PbB 60 μg/100 mL or	
	ALAU 12 mg/L (in 1985)	

biological monitoring at work, setting narrow limits for the use of this concept, it must be recognized that the range of applications of biological indicators is much wider. An excellent example is afforded by the methods currently available for assessing human exposure to carcinogenic and mutagenic agents. An international seminar on this topic, held in December 1983, was organized jointly by the UNEP/ILO/WHO International Programme on Chemical Safety (IPCS), the International Agency for Research on Cancer (IARC), the Commission of the European Communities and the Finnish Institute of Occupational Health[17].

Table 3.7   Lead in air concentration: blood-lead levels and appropriate provisions-sions to be taken

Lead in air concentration $\mu g/L^3$ (time-weighted average over 40 h/week)	PbB level $\mu g\ Pb/$ 100 mL blood	Provision to be taken
40	40	Minimize the risk of lead absorption. Workers be informed.
-	40-50	Regular biological monitoring
75	50	Full application of directive, in particular: - monitoring of lead in air concentration - medical surveillance
150	70	Limit values. Action to be taken in order to minimize exposure.
	70-80	Limit values allowed if other biological parameters are lower than a set limit value. (e.g. ALAU < 20 mg/g creatinine)

The seminar recognized that a certain confusion has existed in distinguishing biological monitoring for exposure from health surveillance, and that the two represent separate components of a continuum which ranges from the measurement of agents in the body to detect exposure, to detection of early signs of disease. A better understanding of the health significance of the biological endpoints measured by these methods is needed before they can be recommended for use in the health surveillance of occupational exposure to carcinogenic and mutagenic agents.

The following methods appear to be those most suited for development and limited use, with appropriate precautions:

- Determination of chemicals and their metabolites in biological fluid and tissues;
- Determination of thioethers in urine;
- Detection of mutagenic activity in urine;

Table 3.8 Determination of ALA in urine by different European laboratories

Samples	Mauzerall and Granick n = 9 Mean ± CV (mg/L)	Davis and Andelman n = 13 Mean ± CV (mg/L)	Grabecki et al. n = 10 Mean ± CV (mg/L)	Wada et al. n = 2 (mg/L)	Kufner et al. n = 1 (mg/L)
A	2.95 ± 28%	4.00 ± 49%	4.68 ± 33%	3.0 1.6	2.1
B	5.59 ± 17%	7.00 ± 24%	7.94 ± 16%	4.8 3.2	5.4
B - A[a]	2.64 ± 17%	3.00 ± 86%	3.26 ± 62%	1.8 1.6	3.3
C	6.20 ± 22%	7.72 ± 18%	8.73 ± 23%	5.3 4.6	6.0
D	15.10 ± 20%	16.57 ± 10%	18.20 ± 18%	13.1 10.8	15.1
D - C[b]	8.90 ± 37%	8.85 ± 26%	9.45 ± 40%	7.8 6.2	9.1

[a] Unsupplemented (A) and supplemented (B) pooled urine samples from persons not occupationally exposed to lead. Expected difference: 3.06 mg ALA/L

[b] Unsupplemented (C) and supplemented (D) pooled urine samples from persons occupationally exposed to lead. Expected difference: 9.97 mg ALA/L

n = number of laboratories reporting.

- Detection of chromosomal aberrations in lymphocytes;
- Detection of sister chromatid exchange in lymphocytes;
- Testing for micronuclei in lymphocytes and/or epithelial cells;
- Determination of sperm morphology (in selected situations).

Practical implementation of these methods must still be undertaken with caution.

It was considered that there was an urgent need to establish a set of criteria by which the methods currently or potentially available could be validated. It was agreed that the factors to be considered in setting such criteria should include the following:

(1) Appropriateness for exposure assessment and health effect assessment;
(2) Results valid for the individual or group;
(3) Reproducibility within and between laboratories;
(4) Accuracy (specificity, recovery);
(5) Detection limit;
(6) Inter- and intra- individual variations in non-exposed reference populations (due to race, sex, age, etc.);
(7) Effects of possible interfering factors (diet, smoking, alcohol, etc.);
(8) Absence of background levels;
(9) Simplicity;
(10) Possibility of sample storage.

Table 3.9 Biological indicators for the assessment of human exposure to industrial chemicals

Compound	Authors	Compound	Authors
Benzene	R Lauwerys	Aluminium	K H Schaller
			H Valentin
Cadmium	L Alessio		
	P Odonc	Chromium	R Franchini
	C Bertelli		A Mutti
	V Foà		B Cavartota
			C Pedroni
Chlorinated	A C Mouster		
hydrocarbon	R L Zielhuis	Copper	A Borghetti
solvents			C Triebig
			K M Schaller
Lead	L Alessio		
	V Foà	Styrene	R Lauwerys
Manganese	H Valentin	Xylene	R Lauwerys
	R Schiele		C Bertelli
			C Cortona
Titanium	H Valentin		P Odonc
	R M Schaller		L Alessio
Toluene	R Lauwerys	Lead Aklyl	L Alessio
			A Dell'Orto
		Mercury	V Foà
Acrylonitrile	C Bertelli		C Bertelli
	A Berlin		
	R Roi	Organo-	H Fallentin
	L Alessio	phosphate	
		pesticides	

Finally it was concluded that it would be desirable to establish, at the international level, the scientific relevance of these methods to provide guidance for researchers and occupational physicians who might be required to provide such information in the workplace. It is strongly emphasized that such information must be given to individuals participating in any epidemiological investigation or monitoring programme.

Currently the Commission of the European Communities, jointly with the WHO and IPCS, is assessing a number of the methods on the basis of the above ten factors and is establishing guidance notes as to the significance of these methods for use at the international level.

PUBLIC HEALTH

In June 1983, the Commission decided to submit to Council a proposal for a directive relating to the protection of dialysis patients by minimization of the exposure to aluminium[18]. The Commission's decision was based upon:

- The continued occurrence of encephalopathy and osteomalacia among dialysis patients;

- The fast-growing number of dialysis patients and the increase in the number of dialysis centres (Table 3.10);

- The increasing amount of travel of persons on dialysis among member states of the European Community;

- The relatively low concern for the aluminium problem among the dialysis centres (Table 3.10);

- A cost estimation of patients' treatment due to complications arising from excess aluminium uptake as compared with aluminium removal and analyses.

Table 3.10   Dialysis patients and aluminium in the European Community

	1971	1977	1979	1981	1983
Number of patients	6,000	25,700	33,800	50,900	55,372 (plus 10,000 in Spain and Portugal)
Dialysis patients/ 1,000,000 inhabitants	--	--	--	190	
Dialysis centres	--	823	933	1,035	1,100 (plus 217 in Spain and Portugal)
Centres analysing for aluminium in serum, water and dialysis fluids	--	--	--	280 (27%)	

Projected number of patients in 1986: 70-75,000, with about 1,400 centres (including Portugal and Spain).

The Commission's proposal covers the following main elements:

- Informing persons in charge of the dialysis centres of the aluminium toxicity problem;

- Limitation of the aluminium level in the dialysis fluids, dialysis concentrates and water used for dilution;
- Regular monitoring of the aluminium levels in the serum of dialysis patients;

- Establishment of reference levels for the aluminium concentration in the plasma (Table 3.11);

- Setting up of a quality assurance programme for aluminium analyses.

Table 3.11 Reference levels for aluminium in plasma of dialysis patients

Level	Comment
> 60 ug/L	Excessive build-up of the body aluminium burden
> 100 µg/L	Appropriate to increase serum aluminium monitoring frequency and health surveillance
200 µg/L	All measures to be taken to ensure that this level is not exceeded in individual patients

Since the transmission of the proposal to Council, the awareness of the aluminium problem has significantly increased among dialysis centres and at the European Pharmacapoeia Commission of the Council of Europe.

It is estimated that in 1986, more than 0.25 million aluminium analyses will be performed in the European Community. The Commission is particularly pleased with the IUPAC efforts to develop reference methods. The quality assurance programme mentioned before will be set up this year.

CONCLUSIONS

The interest in introducing biological parameters to the legislative framework (directives and recommendations) of the European Communities has grown extensively over the past decade. This paper has concentrated on the use of these parameters in the framework of routine monitoring.

We are of course aware of the considerable expansion which has taken place in the research context and encourage it to achieve future monitoring tools.

In our opinion, the current legislation should generate yearly more than one million analyses for clearly identified, specific purposes in occupational and public health, all requiring severe quality control which we promote and encourage.

REFERENCES

1. Recht P, Smeets J, Amavis R and Berlin A, Quality Control and Harmonisation Programmes for the Assessment of Environmental Pollution in the European Communities. Proceedings of the EPA-WHO International Conference on Environmental Sensing and Assessment. (Las Vegas: 1975).

2. Berlin A, Wolff AH and Hasegawa Y, (eds). (1979). The Use of Biological Specimens for the Assessment of Human Exposure to Environmental Pollutants. (Martinus Nijhoff: Boston, The Hague).

3. Council Directive of 29 March 1977 on biological screening of the population for lead. Official J Eur Communities, L 105, 10.

4. Berlin A and Schaller KH, (1974). European standardized method for the determination of delta-aminolevulinic acid dehydratase activity in blood. Klin Chem Klin Biochem 12, 389-390.

5. Berlin A, (1982). Assessment of exposure to lead of the general population in the European Community through biological monitoring. Environ Monit Assess, 2, 225-231.

6. Berlin A, Yodaiken RE and Henman BA, (eds). (1984). Assessment of Toxic Agents at the Workplace: Roles of Ambient and Biological Monitoring. (Martinus Nijhoff: Boston, The Hague).

7. Berlin A, Yodaiken RE and Logan DC, (1982). International seminar on the assessment of toxic agents at the workplace: roles of ambient and biological monitoring. Int Arch Occup Environ Hlth, 50, 197-207.

8. WHO Technical Report Series 647, (1980). Recommended Health-Based Limits in Occupational Exposure to Heavy Metals. (Geneva).

9. WHO Technical Report Series 664, (1981). Recommended Health-Based Limits in Occupational Exposure to Selected Organic Solvents. (Geneva).

10. WHO Technical Report Series 677, (1982). Recommended Health-Based Limits in Occupational Exposure to Pesticides. (Geneva).

11. Council Directive (EEC/605/82) of July 1982 on the protection of workers from harmful exposure to metallic lead and its ionic compounds at work. Official J Eur Communities, L 247, 12.

12. Proposal for a Council Directive on the protection of workers from harmful exposure to metallic lead and its ionic compounds at work. Official J Eur Communities, C 324. (23.12.1979).

13. Davis JR and Andelman SL, (1967). Urinary delta-aminolevulinic acid levels in lead poisoning. A modified method for the rapid determination of urinary delta-aminolevulinic acid using disposable ion-exchange chromatographic columns. Arch Environ Hlth, 15, 53-59.

14. Berlin A and Smeets J, (1974). European intercomparison programmes and harmonization of techniques with special reference to heavy metals in biological fluids. Presented at the 4th Annual Symposium on Record Advances on the Analytical Chemistry of Pollutants, June, Basle.

15. Alessio L, Berlin A, Roi R and Boni M, (eds). (1983). Human Biological Monitoring of Industrial Chemicals Series. EUR 8476 EN. (Luxembourg, Ispra).

16. Alessio L, Berlin A, Boni M and Roi R, (eds). (1984). Biological Indicators for the Assessment of Human Exposure to Industrial Chemicals. EUR 8903 EN. (Luxembourg, Ispra).

17. Berlin A, Draper M, Hemminki K and Vainio H, (1984). International seminar on methods of monitoring human exposure to Carcinogenic and mutagenic agents. Int Arch Occup Environ Hlth, 54, 369-375.

18. Proposal for a Council Directive relating to the protection of dialysis patients by minimizing the exposure to aluminium. Official J Eur Communities, C 202, 5.

4

Current Economic, Technical and Political Pressures at the Laboratory Level: Some Benefits Towards Health Care Delivery

JG Lines and N Sanders

INTRODUCTION

The original title for this paper referred only to political, economic and technical pressures and it would have been almost natural to strike a pessimistic note on account of the various anxieties expressed by those involved in health care delivery. However there are considerable benefits to be gained as a result of the present economic and political climate including not only the provision of better health care for the community but also more job satisfaction for laboratory staff and better use of financial resources.

This paper will consider only one way of working towards such benefits, but it is a way which is justifiable in ECCLS circles because it could lead to the suggestion of a subject for another paper standard, namely a standard on laboratory facts and figures or what may preferably be called management data. To show how these economic, political and technical pressures can be turned to advantage, a few recent experiences are presented from our own health district which was formerly a very deprived area in terms of clinical laboratory facilities.

THE NEED FOR RELIABLE MANAGEMENT INFORMATION

Several years ago, it was clear that considerable pressure would be put on the laboratories of the health care industry to become more efficient than hitherto in terms of providing a service (both in providing what was required and in not providing what was inessential), and also in terms of being financially more efficient. We felt that the best way to respond to these pressures, would be to have available as detailed as possible a database of factual information on workload, costing, productivity, quality assurance data, etc. Consequently records were kept of the precise number not just of patient samples analysed, but also of the numbers of assays which had to be processed for instrument calibration and for quality assurance purposes etc. The exact costs of individual tests were determined by dividing the total price of invoices for reagents and other consumables for a particular test, by the number of patient test results obtained.

It is not the purpose of this paper to discuss how such data can bring or have brought about major changes in laboratory practice, but to deal with the 'fine-tuning' which is possible when quality data are available, and the way in which it has led to those benefits mentioned earlier.

Let us first consider a simple example of fine-tuning which can save unnecessary waste of money on laboratory consumables. About 15 months ago, it was possible to persuade our local administration to top up a regional grant for a large selective analyser so that, instead of the model being offered, a superior model could be obtained. For those not familiar with the UK system, major capital equipment is normally purchased by regional (or county) health authorities and not by the local (or district) health authority. The case for purchasing the superior model was that it would be considerably cheaper to run as well as having technical advantages.

Having succeeded in getting the superior model, it was felt that the claims of it being cheaper to run should be investigated as a part of maintaining our 'credibility rating' (see below). Expectations and actual experience did not always coincide. For example, in the case of creatinine it was more expensive than anticipated, but we had had a similar experience three years earlier with the same test on the G300 and had eventually identified the cause as a leaking pump causing reagent wastage - indeed it was the cause of this difference and when corrected led to a cost saving. In other cases we did better than expected by maximizing the use of reagents before their expiry times, whereas with other tests, particularly enzyme assays, there were higher test costs than anticipated because of the expiry of unstable reagents. The pack sizes will therefore be changed to minimize wastage and save costs. Although it might be said that this is only fine-tuning, today laboratories have to be in the fine tuning business to respond to demands being made. In any case, the total amount saved can be quite considerable over a 12 month period.

THE IMPORTANCE OF A HIGH CREDIBILITY RATING

There are two types of credibility ratings which readily spring to mind. The obvious one is the way in which our clinical colleagues look at the service we provide. However, more relevant to the theme of this seminar is the credibility which laboratory workers have in the eyes of their financial and administrative masters for the way in which they run the service - or perhaps more importantly, their private view on the validity of claims from the laboratory for more resources.

It is our belief that merely having available in the laboratory quality data on test costs - or any other quality data - is only of limited value, but if the data is made generally available, it begins to reap benefits.   For example, bringing information on test costs to the attention of clinicians may well influence the pattern of requesting - anecdotal evidence suggests that it does but that will not be discussed here.   Bringing that same information to the attention of administrative colleagues most certainly makes them aware that the laboratory does take financial matters seriously, and providing that the information is reliable the credit rating of the laboratory goes up.

There are two principal routes by which we regularly disseminate information about laboratory services and their costs. One is the publication of an extensive departmental annual report each year and the other is an occasional newsletter - **Biosek** (Biochemistry News for South East Kent) - in which key messages are presented.   Both the annual report and **Biosek** are distributed very widely as a deliberate policy and it is clear from comments received that both get read and have contributed towards establishing credence.

This recently paid off in an unexpected and record way. Following the sudden withdrawal of a free national service for IgE and common allergens, this service had to be provided locally. The request for funding was made on a Monday afternoon, tabled at the meeting of the executive administrative group (the district management team) the next morning and approved.   This probably approaches a national record for speed in successfully applying for recurring revenue monies - but our track record in validity of claims was said to be an important factor.   Thus it constitutes a benefit in our formulation of requests in response to the pertaining economic and political climate.

THE IMPACT OF TECHNICAL ADVANCES

Selective analysis

The relative merits of the blockbuster screening/profiling approach versus selective laboratory investigation will not be debated. However the results of the regular preaching of the 'gospel of selectivity' on laboratory workload and ultimately the budget will be considered and it will be shown how this can lead to both greater job satisfaction and the maximum use of limited financial resources.

We have been able reliably to assess the effects of having available a selective analyser because the health district for which we provide the clinical chemistry services has two hospitals 40 km apart, each with their own laboratory.   All same-day turnaround tests are done at both laboratories,   but specialized (or less urgent) tests are done at only one or other laboratory.   The workload and staffing are almost identical in the two laboratories and the consultant physicians and surgeons work at both hospitals.

However, the difference between the hospitals is that at the William Harvey Hospital a selective analyser (Greiner G300)   was installed in December 1980 whereas Buckland Hospital,   Dover worked with non-selective equipment until one year ago.   Table 4.1 presents the average test/request ratio for the five years to March

Table 4.1 Test/request ratios in two hospitals in South East Kent

	Buckland Hospital	William Harvey Hospital
1980-81	5.51	5.29
1981-82	5.53	4.38 ─Selective
1982-83	6.05	3.66
1983-84	6.22	3.47 ▼
1984-85	4.67 ─Selective ▼	3.17

1985 (the test/request ratio is the average number of individual tests that are asked for on each blood sample).

At the William Harvey Hospital the test/request ratio was found to drop year by year whereas at Dover it remained fairly constant – the small increase between 1981/82 and 1982/83 was due to removal of radioimmunoassay (with a low test/request ratio) from Dover to the William Harvey Hospital – and accounts for some of the drop there in the same period. Notice particularly though the final fifth year – there is a continuing decrease in the William Harvey figure, and within only nine months of getting a selective analyser at Buckland (a Greiner G400), their test/request ratio dropped by 24.9%. Had there not been this drop, 50,268 unwanted tests would have been carried out at a cost of about £7500 on what is really a very small workload (32,000 requests annually). Whilst this cost-saving was brought about partly by the change in analytical equipment , the recent year-by-year cost-saving that is represented by the drop in test/request ratio at the William Harvey Hospital is purely a reflection of changed practice in requesting by clinicians – brought about, we believe, by our efforts at education through **Biosek** etc.

This cost-saving has led to improved job satisfaction and a much wider use of our limited financial allocation. Our own health authority operates a type of 'reward' incentive scheme to encourage cost-saving, such that budgets are not greatly lowered on account of identifiable cost-saving (at least 60% of any saving is automatically returned to the budget holder for use as he wishes). It was possible to use the 'selectivity' saving to fund the provision of a much-needed therapeutic drug monitoring service and also to provide the quality of specific protein service which is expected in 1985. Of course providing such services gave every one more interest in their work and created the need to learn new skills (not just technical ones but also interpretive skills). These led to an inevitable improvement in job satisfaction which, together with the wider and better clinical service which the laboratory can now offer, provide an interesting commentary on benefits which have arisen as a direct result of our responding positively to the pertaining economic pressures.

The cost of producing the report

Let us look at another way in which technical advances - together with the pertaining economic and political climates - may influence the way in which clinical chemistry (and perhaps other disciplines) laboratories work.

Although an important aspect of overall cost-effectiveness is how useful a test result is in patient management, this will not be considered here. What is of concern is the cost of producing patient reports and the relative costs of producing reports from different sections of the clinical laboratory. The four principal cost elements involved in the production of a report (Table 4.2) are as follows:

- **Capital costs** which may be amortized over 8 years;

- **Annual maintenance contracts** on equipment. These are usually 7-10% of the capital cost;

- **Salaries** of technical staff. For setting these costs we prefer to take the salary of a qualified technician with about five years' experience quoting not just the salary received but the total cost to the employer (including superannuation, national insurance etc.);

- **Reagent costs** which may be expressed in terms of patient reports. They may be derived by multiplying the average cost of reagents for one test by the average test/request ratio for patient reports. This is approximately 4.2 for reports from the main area of the laboratory and it might include electrolytes, urea, glucose or liver function tests etc.

If we look at the main laboratory area and consider the use, for example, of the Greiner G300 selective analyser, we have a capital cost of £56,000 amortized to £7000 per annum. The cost of reagents for the average test is 10 pence and working unhurriedly one technician can produce 1800 reports a week, each of which would have between 4 and 5 test results on it. Thus, the average cost is 63 pence per report.

In radioimmunoassay, although the cost of equipment is less and the cost of maintenance much less, the productivity of a technician in terms of reports is below 10% of that of someone working a large analyser, and each report normally has only one or two results on it. Reagents are much more expensive, particularly as many radioimmunoassays have to be done in duplicate, and there is a slightly higher proportion of standards and controls in relation to patient sample assays than for G300 work. The final result is that an endocrine report coming from the radioimmunoassay section of the laboratory costs approximately £3 to produce.

Table 4.2   Report production costs

Equipment capital costs, amortized over 8 years: annual cost = E

Equipment maintenance: annual cost = M

One technician's salary   annually = S
(+ social security contributions, superannuation, etc.)

Reagent consumption   annually = R
(by one technician working 37 h/wk, 52 wk/y

$$\text{Cost of 1 report} = \frac{E + M + S + R}{\text{reports/annum}}$$

In terms of the effects of technology on laboratory practice, let us consider the immunochemistry section of the laboratory, that is carrying out specific protein assays, drug assays for therapeutic drug monitoring and possibly some endocrinology. Our experience with the manual Beckman ICS system is that technician productivity is about 1000 test results per week at a patient report cost of about half that using radioimmunoassay. It is this sort of cost analysis data together with the economic climate in which we are all working that may well herald a change in our working methods.

CONCLUSIONS

Whilst we all know that we are working in a somewhat stricter and more pressing economic and political atmosphere, by addressing ourselves to some details which we have often ignored previously, we can discover some interesting facts. It is possible that the present climate is actually more beneficial than damaging in terms of producing a more efficient and effective clinical laboratory serv-ice. Perhaps ECCLS should consider establishing a standard for management statistics in clinical laboratory practice.

Part 2

THE CLINICAL LABORATORY IN THE CHANGING SCENE OF HEALTH CARE

5

The Clinical Laboratory in the Changing Scene of Health Care as Seen by a Professional Society Member

M Roth

INTRODUCTION

Clinical laboratories are presently facing a number of problems caused by the trends of modern health care. Among the most relevant three particular trends may be identified.

(1)   **Increasing service from the laboratory.** Many new tests have become available in recent years, and physicians are ordering a lot of some of them. Emergency laboratories capable of providing fast service are much appreciated by physicians, who desire the extension of such services.

(2)   **Reduction of costs.** Many new tests are expensive. For some of them, the benefit to the patient is not such that it would justify the increased cost. Political authorities and administrations are concerned with the rising cost of medicine, and they tend to impose budgetary restrictions which may limit the development of laboratories.

(3)   **By-passing of professional laboratories through the development of simplified tests.** Technological advances have resulted in the development of simplified analytical tests that can be performed outside the laboratories, for example in wards, doctor's offices, or even at the patient's home. The advantage of such tests is that they are very convenient to perform. Whether or not their quality and cost are acceptable, they represent a challenge to the professional laboratory.

In response to these various trends, professional laboratories have to redefine their attitude and the characteristics of their activity.

TRENDS TOWARDS INCREASING SERVICE FROM THE LABORATORY

It is clear that fast execution and reporting of analyses is becoming an important requisite for laboratories. One reason is that in hospitals the daily cost per patient has increased enormously, so that one tries to reduce the period of stay of patients as much as possible. If the laboratory works fast and the reports are available early, then many waiting times are eliminated. Another reason is the necessity for emergency admission units to determine rapidly whether a patient requires hospitalization or may be sent back home. A good emergency laboratory is essential for that purpose.

To achieve the necessary speed, one has not only to use fast analysers, but also to make sure that no time is lost during the transport of the samples and the transmission of results to the doctors.

Laboratories are therefore interested in the development of well-organized systems for the taking of samples and their transport. In hospitals it is possible, under certain conditions, to use pneumatic tube devices for the transport of samples for chemistry, and for the dispatching of results. In the laboratory a part of the work previously done by automatic batch analyses will be taken over by fast selective analysers working in the profile mode. For the fast transmission of results, different ways may be considered. One may either send reports printed in the laboratory to the doctors by the fastest physical route available, such as pneumatic post system, or use a computer system capable of formatting the results to make them available on ward terminals. What should be avoided is transcription of results by handwriting or keyboard typing, as this introduces human error and represents a loss of time. The best solution is represented by a laboratory computer connected directly or indirectly to terminals that may be consulted by the doctors.

In recent years, a number of new analyses have been requested by clinicians. These include the analyses of drugs, new hormones, receptors, new viruses and new serological tests. The techniques are often quite sophisticated. Laboratories have to adapt themselves to this new situation by acquiring the necessary expertise.

TRENDS TOWARDS REDUCTION IN COSTS

The second problem laboratories are faced with is that of reduction of costs, or at least control of cost increase. A practical manifestation of the problem is represented by budgets severely limited by the administrations. A laboratory manager will always try to cope with a limited budget by taking measures for increasing the working efficiency of the personnel, and for making economies in the purchase of apparatus and reagents. It may be anticipated that in coming years the choice of instruments and methods will be influenced by the cost of the associated reagents and consumables. Black-box instruments with locked-in chemistries are considered with suspicion by laboratory people, who will whenever possible give preference to reagents subject to free competition. It is true that some systems for which it is compulsory to buy both the instrument and the consumables from the same manufacturer work quite well. However, customers are not prepared to pay any price for running such instruments, especially if these are in competition with other machines accommodating cheaper reagents.

A consequence of the fact that laboratories try to reduce expenses due to reagents is that industry now offers automatic analysers capable of working with very small amounts of reagents. This has become an important selling argument.

Whatever measures are taken by laboratories to reduce running costs, there is a limit below which either the quality or the quantity of analyses will have to be reduced. Under stringent budgetary limitations, the response of laboratories will normally consist of an adaptation of the number of analyses done to the available budget. Analytical accounting systems are now in favour even in state administrations, and there is a tendency to run state laboratories in the same way as private ones, namely on cost-per-test basis, and on virtual bills calculated for every clinic from which analyses are ordered.

Laboratory scientists are progressively turning into managers. Management represents an aspect of their activity for which they were not necessarily prepared during their studies. Here again, an adaptation is necessary.

THE BY-PASSING OF PROFESSIONAL LABORATORIES

The third problem concerns the very essence of the professional laboratory, and resides in the fact that analytical methods are now offered by industry with the claim that they may be performed even by non-professionals. Such methods include dry chemistry systems, in which an analytical reaction is performed on a solid support and a product is measured by reflectance or fluorimetry. One may ask three important questions regarding such simplified tests:

When compared to the same tests done in the specialized laboratory, are they:

> more convenient?
> more reliable?
> more economical?

Generally speaking these tests are more convenient to the user, but it is admitted that many of them are less reliable, at least in the hands of non-qualified personnel, and that they cost more. The role of laboratories in this respect is to make sure that these tests are evaluated with objectivity by those who use the results. Laboratories will also try to demonstrate, in the cases where this applies, that they work more reliably and economically.

CONCLUSIONS

Having tried to define the various and often conflicting forces that interact at the boundary between the laboratory and its environment, it is worthwhile to consider the presumable outcome of this complex interaction.

It is inevitable that the efficiency with which laboratories are working will be the subject of increased scrutiny from administrations. It is also inevitable that some of the analyses previously made by centralized laboratories will move to the bedside, the doctor's office or the patient's home. This will not necessarily mean that laboratories will have to reduce their personnel or to work less, because on the other hand new demands, such as fast responses and additional tests, are made by the physicians.

The best way laboratories can respond to the changing scene of health care is to adapt themselves, so as to play a different role in a new scene.

6

The Clinical Laboratory in the Changing Scene of Health Care as Seen by an Industry Member

JE Barclay

This paper highlights some potential problems which may affect the pace of advancement of clinical laboratory science. These problems may be more readily appreciated by laboratory professionals who have an international outlook on medicine, technology and regulatory affairs.

INTRODUCTION

Industry has become the source of innovation for most new laboratory technology. Fewer and fewer laboratory professionals are free to develop new analytical techniques or procedures as in former times. For analytical technologies involving chemists, engineers, software specialists, hydraulics experts etc, few academic institutions have the required mixture of staff expertise or financial support to allow them to make developments beyond feasibility stages. This traditional role has largely been replaced by one of evaluation and clinical validation of tests, procedures and equipment which have been developed by industry, and a new form of partnership is emerging.

Industry can only afford to conduct basic research if the industry is profitable. Profit is necessary because a high technology company must invest 10-15% of its earnings in research and development in order to come up (hopefully) with new products on a regular basis. High technology products take longer and longer, and cost more and more to develop. Once developed, their commercial lifespan is shorter and shorter.

There is a threat to the pace of advancement of clinical laboratory science which lies in the possible application of cost containment and regulatory procedures inappropriately focussed in the clinical laboratory field. The clinical laboratory is only one part of health care delivery. World-wide sales of clinical laboratory products have been estimated at only 6 per cent of health care expenditure[1].

The role of government agencies is of great importance, and

will become even more so. In some countries a slowing down or even cessation of some types of research may already be taking place, due to the high cost of developing data required for regulatory approval procedures originally conceived for pharmaceutical products.

CLINICAL LABORATORY SCIENCE IN HEALTH CARE DELIVERY

Health care delivery

The health status of any community is greatly influenced by genetic and biological factors, as well as social factors such as alcohol, drugs, smoking and accidents (Figure 6.1).

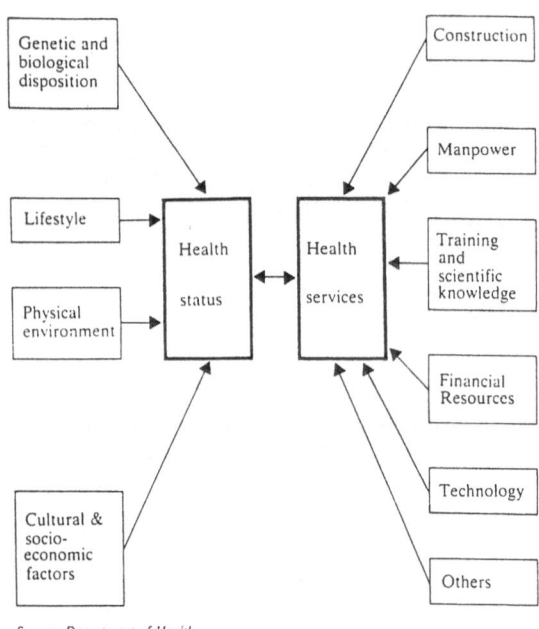

Source: Department of Health

Figure 6.1 The Health 2000 report model.

Clinical laboratory science is a branch of medicine in which the laboratory examination of body fluids and tissues contributes to patient care. It has several components:

- The development of methods of analysis;
- Applications of analytical methods to new analytes;
- The interpretation of results, including collecting databases for developing reference values;
- Establishing the usefulness and clinical validity of tests or test strategies.

Figure 6.1 does not suggest how financial and other resources should be allocated. The allocation to the clinical laboratory will probably reflect the type of care provided in hospitals, and this in turn will depend on levels of:

- Health education;
- Preventive medicine;
- Community care for the disabled, elderly, mentally and chronically sick.

Clinical laboratory science will evolve with new medical knowledge and the development of new technologies. These new technologies may be for use within the laboratory and also outside e.g. imaging or scanning techniques which replace in vitro methods of diagnosis.

Clinical laboratory science: demand led or technology driven?

Professor Adam Fleck of the New Charing Cross Hospital in London attempted an analysis of the historical evolution of laboratory testing. On a time axis (Figure 6.2) he put:

- Medical and physiological discoveries;
- Analytical techniques;
- Developments in electronics and in computing;
- The appearance of automated analysers;
- The introduction of professional societies;
- The introduction of external quality control schemes.

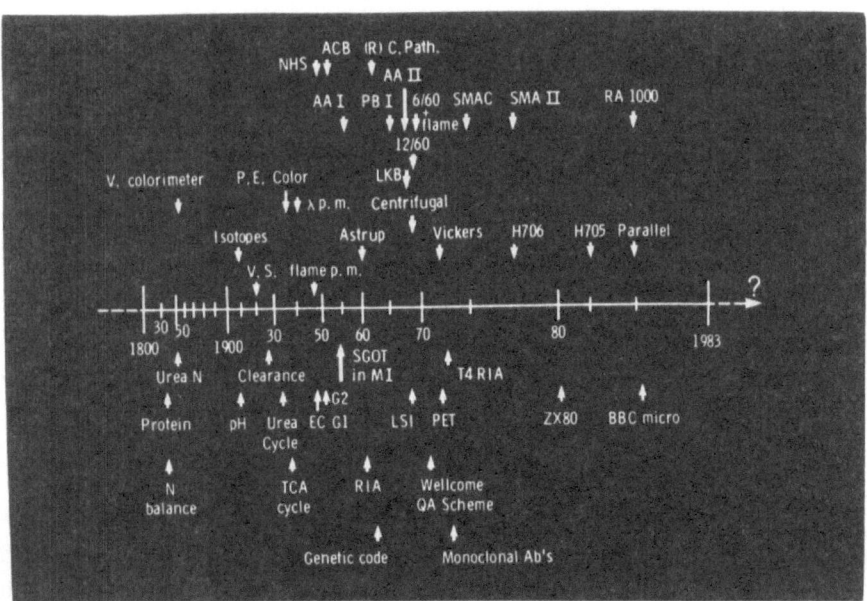

Figure 6.2 Clinical laboratory science: demand-led or technology driven? (Reproduced with permission of Professor Fleck)

In annual reports from pathologists in the 1920s and 1930s there were already comments on the ever increasing workload of pathology specimens.   In the 1950s and 1960s the clinical laboratory was revolutionized by the introduction of automation, first with the single channel autoanalyser and later the 6 and 12 channel SMA systems.   At the same time the number of biochemistry tests showed an enormous growth.

An obvious development has been the constant trend to the industrialization of reagent manufacture.   Automation allowed the laboratory to cope with the growth, to increase technician productivity and to reduce greatly the cost per test (Table 6.1).   Although the cost per test was reduced, the overall costs increased. The cost escalation brought the laboratory to the attention of health administrators and government.

Table 6.1 Montefiore and Albert Einstein Laboratory: impact of automation. From Ref.3 reproduced with permission

	1965	1975	Change
Inpatients served	13,318	22,740	1.7x
Outpatients serviced	60,151	234,192	3.9x
Tests performed	214,000	2,213,000	10.3x
Budget	$562,000	$1,126,000	2.0x
Budget in 1965	$562,000	$ 624,000	1.1x
Cost per test in 1965	$ 2.63	$ 0.29	9.1x less
Results to floor	5:00 PM	12:00 Noon	5 hours earlier

The number of inpatients almost doubled in this period, and the number of out-patients quadrupled. The number of tests increased more than ten-fold. Not only were total laboratory costs held to 1965 levels, but also, patient care was improved by the large increase in the laboratory information that was made available. The new laboratory equipment is an important tool for the early detection of disease. While it is enormously difficult to quantify the exact value of the patient care benefits provided by the improved data on the patients' well-being, there is little doubt of this value which adds further justification for the investment in this cost-reducing automation.

When medical discovery has added a new analyte to the laboratory science repertoire, there have been three historical phases of evolution:

-       first a manual assay (research),
-       then a commercial kit,
-       then an automated instrument.

Increasingly, and largely as a result of the application of technologies to the simplification of analytical procedures, there is a tendency to go directly from research methods to automated analytical devices.

Professor Fleck concluded that the growth in testing was

both technology driven and demand led[4].

FUTURE EXPECTATIONS

Emerging technology

Others have reviewed future laboratory technology more completely[5,6], but there are some important features on instrumentation that should be mentioned briefly and selectively.

(1) Electronics and EDP Analytical systems need to be reliable, and will use well-proven components.

-   With 16 bit computers, response times are very fast. Automated analysers will increasingly feature distributed microprocessors with 'intelligent' samplers and other peripheral devices.
-   Self-checking diagnostics and remote checking of instruments via modem will become commonplace.
-   Low cost memory devices will be used to store reference values, perform QC checks and perhaps even to make diagnostic interpretation.
-   Curve smoothing techniques and automatic calculation are commonplace today. Sophisticated mathematical approaches to response-curve analysis will be used to eliminate analytical interferences and reduce the need for re-calibration and control.

(2) Bio-sensors and ion-selective electrodes Despite a decade of development, ion selective semiconductors in the form of ISFET or Chemfet are not much closer to commercial reality. Problems of encapsulation and instability are likely to persist, and to prevent their use in instruments, although not for short term in vitro work.

For routine analyses, only sodium and potassium electrodes are fast enough for high capacity analysers

(3) Optics Conventional spectrophotometers are difficult to mechanize and may require relatively large liquid volumes. Simplified diode and diode-array optics will be used to reduce hardware costs, although some of these devices are highly sophisticated. These devices are really 'calibrated read-stations' for light absorption, rather than colorimeters.

(4) Fluid transfer technology The simple advances, such as putting simultaneous multitest capability on a centrifugal analyser, have already been done. More tablet, slide and other dry chemistry formulations will appear, in addition to those we already know. The 'zero carryover' approach to wet chemistry using Teflon sample and reagent probes, coupled with selective wetting by fluorocarbon oil, is well known[7]. We can expect further refinements permitting use of very low volumes of sample and reagent.

(5) Ligand assays These will be increasingly developed in solid phase or strip form even for low level analytes such as peptide hormones or tumour markers. Applications of monoclonal antibodies to microbiology will compete with the use of DNA probes for viral and bacterial identification. Assays for new substances such as cell growth factors will be developed.

More sensitive labelling techniques will appear, involving enhancement of colour development or luminescence. These new techniques may allow sensitive assays to be simply incorporated into conventional chemistry analysers.

What are the foreseeable medical demands?

Medical demand is a complex issue, varying according to the population under study, medical practice including availability and use of pharmaceuticals, and local reimbursement or health insurance schemes.

(1) The third world On a worldwide basis, the most significant changes in medical demand for laboratory services will come from the emergence of the third world. The population growth in industrialized countries is around 1%, going from around 1.1 billion today to 1.3 billion in the year 2000.

In the developing countries, growth is over 2% per annum and the population growth will be 9 times greater - 2 billion more people requiring medical care[8].

The types of pharmaceutical care and laboratory testing needed here are quite different from those in the industrialized world. There will be a need for basic biochemistry and haematology combined with tests for infectious and parasitic diseases.

(2) The elderly In the industrialized world the rising prevalence of the elderly is already changing the pattern of testing[9]. The number of people over 65 years of age will not change very much over the next 25 years, but there will be a 7% increase in the number aged 75-85 and a 34% increase in those aged over 85 years. People aged over 85 are 10-14 times more likely to be resident in hospital than those aged 65-69[10].

This is a two sided problem - apart from the increased cost of health care of the elderly, there will be proportionally fewer workers paying taxes to pay for them. The rising proportion of elderly brings about a growth in testing for cancer and for chronic and degenerative diseases.

The effect on patterns of testing in hospitals will depend on where long term care takes place (home, hospital or other institution).

(3) New forms of treatment may alter patterns of laboratory testing Cimetidine was developed in the 1970s, and it is an example of a drug which not only revolutionized patient management, but also resulted in a major reduction of a specific part of the laboratory workload. Surgical costs were reduced by 40%, and with the

reduction in vagotomy and pyloroplasty operations came a corresponding decrease in electrolyte assays.

In the next few years we can expect some new types of drug to emerge, particularly in the fields of cancer management, immune modifiers and anti-inflammatory compounds.

How will technology meet future demands?

The overriding factors will be economic, both from the point of view of government in allocating resources, and from industry in developing products.

New approaches to resource allocation will be developed. The exponential growth in laboratory testing in the 1960s and 1970s led to different ways of limiting the increase. The details vary from country to country, but the main approaches have been:

(1) **Ceilings on capital expenditure.** Above a certain level, the laboratory must apply to a local, regional or national committee for approval of investment.

(2) **Ceilings on annual expenditures.** The laboratory operates within a fixed budget. Introduction of new tests must be accompanied by reductions in the numbers or costs of existing ones. The budget may be fixed directly or via insurance reimbursement.

(3) **Workload/staff ratios.** Some countries have regulations giving staffing levels for a given workload (as measured by an arbitrary system). Labour costs are 60-80% of the laboratory budget and so this type of regulation has the dual function of maintaining employment levels in the community and limiting capital available for investment in equipment.

(4) **Diagnosis related groups (DRGs).** Of all the procedures for controlling laboratory expenditures, the US introduction of DRGs (Diagnosis related groups) is perhaps the most far reaching. The concept is easily understood (see Chapter 8) and is likely to be adopted in other countries.

It is easy to see how these cost-containment measures may, by delaying capital expenditures, not only delay the introduction of new tests or techniques, especially if they are innovative, within the hospital laboratory or for use in the community, but also require a restructuring of organization. In the next ten years, it is probable that new accounting and cost management techniques will be brought into health care and into the laboratory, allowing full scope for administrators and laboratory directors to be truly cost effective in health care delivery.

In this respect ECCLS is already working on a cost analysis standard for use within the laboratory.

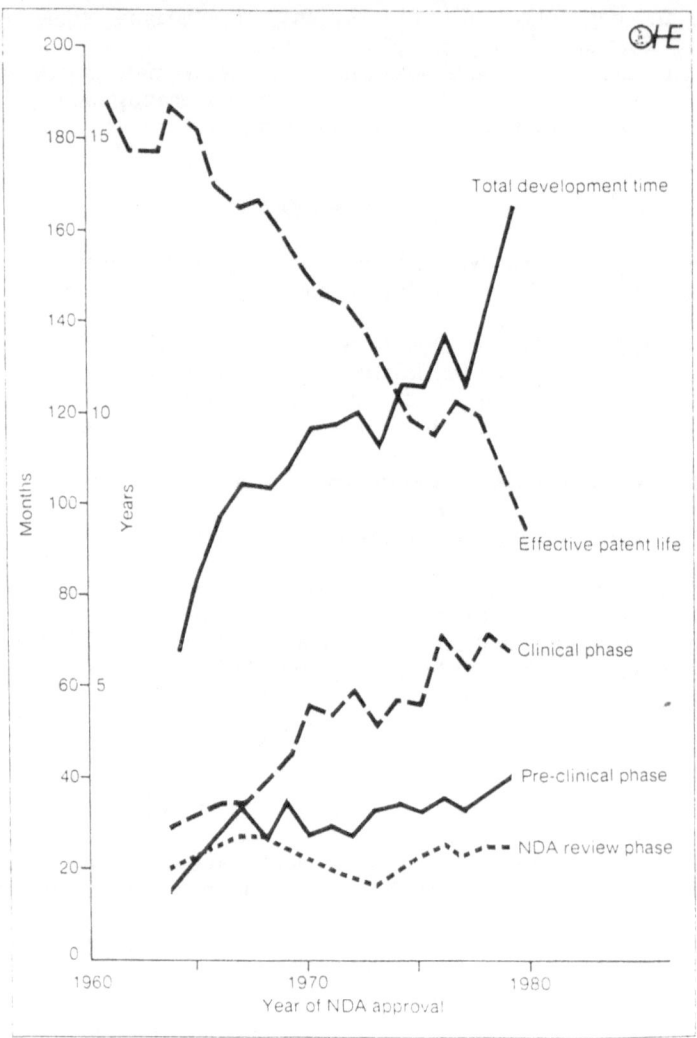

**Figure 6.3   The development time of US marketed drugs.
Reproduced with permission**

HOW QUICKLY CAN TECHNOLOGY RESPOND TO A DEMAND?

Considering once more the experience of the pharmaceutical industry[11], Figure 6.3 shows the ever increasing time taken to develop a drug (which means ever increasing costs) coupled with the steady fall in effective patent life. Nearly all of the increase in development time is due to an increase in the clinical phase of testing which is necessary to comply with various regulatory requirements for proof and efficacy.

For this reason patent laws relating to pharmaceuticals in the United States were recently given a seven year extension.

52

The length of time taken to develop new techniques is also increasing. Published patents show that sometimes more than 10 years of fundamental technology research can be required. The same types of regulation which affect innovative products have been applied to the diagnostics and medical equipment field. Particularly when considering the United States, small companies may not be able to afford to develop new diagnostic tests in specialized areas of medicine because of the length of time (and cost) of introduction. There are recent examples of companies coming to Europe, where they can pursue research, develop clinical validity data and bring a product to market faster than in their own regulated homeland.

These are all areas in which government may play an important role.

HOW DOES INDUSTRY REACT TO THESE ECONOMIC AND REGULATORY PHENOMENA?

Industry is looking to industry

There is an increasing cooperation and joint development between companies with complementary skills and technologies. Every month there are reports in the trade press of new joint ventures, often on very specific projects.

Industry is looking to the profession

More and more, academic clinical laboratories will be involved with fundamental developments and applications of technology. Professionals will once again be consulted early in commercial development plans, and the developments made so as to make it easier to carry out field trials of early prototype instruments or model reagent systems.

Industry is looking to government

In some countries, e.g. Japan, there will be a change in the way in which introduction of laboratory products will be regulated. The revised procedure will be more relevant to laboratory requirements. Industry looks to governments to apply logical procedures which avoid unnecessary duplication of validation studies or documentation.

Industry is looking to standards organizations

There is a need today to rationalize the various national preferred methods in clinical chemistry, although the recommendation by scientific organizations of patented techniques in clinical chemistry is still in debate.

There will be an even greater need in future for a broad international view to standardization of procedures and for reference preparations in the emerging fields of tumour specific antigens and immune modulators etc. Assays for these may need to be compared by professional societies, perhaps via workshops as were used for tissue typing antigens, and are currently being held for lymphocyte surface markers.

In short, industry looks to standards organizations for a rational approach to technology assessment.

CONCLUSION

Perhaps through full and mutual understanding between government, the professions and industry, it will be possible to avoid unnecessary constraints on innovation. By providing a forum for discussion, ECCLS can encourage and simplify the development of new technologies and help further the evolution of clinical laboratory science.

REFERENCES

1. Little A D,(1980). International health care strategies for the 1980s: diversification or specialisation. Impact.
2. Summary Outline of the Health 2000 Report. (1984). The Netherlands Department of Health, The Hague, The Netherlands.
3. Whitehead E C, (1981). A Plan For Cost Containment. Statement before the Subcommittee on Health and the Environment Committee on Interstate and Foreign Commerce. (Technicon Instruments Corporation, New York).
4. Fleck A, (1984). Technicon Seminar on Clinical Chemistry Analysis - Continuous Flow or Discrete? (Wilmslow, UK).
5. Broughton P M G, Carter T N and Clark P M S, (1983). Instrumentation. Clin. Biochem., 16, 317-329.
6. Stinshoff K E, Freytag J W, Laska P F and Gill-Pazaris L. (1985). Clinical Chemistry. Anal. Chem., 57, 114R-130R.
7. Smith J, Svenjak D, Turrell J and Vlastelica D (1982). An Innovative Technology for 'Random Access Sampling'. Clin. Chem., 28, 1867-1872.
8. Nowotny O, (1982). Europe: the Economic Challenge. In Wells N (ed.) The Second Pharmaceutical Revolution (London: Office of Health Economics).
9. Davies S, (1984). 1984: A Year of Major Change. Clinica, 126, 12-13.
10. Andrews K, (1985). Leader. Br. Med. J., 290, 1023-1024.
11. Wardell W, (1982). Discussion. In Wells N (ed.) The Second Pharmaceutical Revolution, p. 106. (London: Office of Health Economics).

7

The Clinical Laboratory in the Changing Scene of Health Care as Seen by a Health Agency Member

R Netter

A discussion about the contribution of the clinical laboratory sciences might seem incongruous in 1985 in view of their dramatic development in industrialized countries. However, procedures are becoming increasingly automated and require careful standardization to enhance their value and comparability.

CLINICAL LABORATORY SCIENCE - WHICH?

The clinical laboratory sciences have a wide impact on the population as a whole.

(1)   Clinical laboratory procedures are practised throughout life.

-     Before marriage tests for syphilis and rubella may be carried out;
-     During pregnancy immunological testing for disease such as toxoplasmosis may be appropriate as may the testing of amniotic fluid or foetal blood samples for the detection of congenital abnormalities of the foetus;
-     Screening the newborn for treatable diseases such as congenital hypothyroidism and phenylketonuria has considerably improved the outlook for affected patients;
-     Laboratory tests are used for making or confirming clinical diagnoses, monitoring recovery and for the adjustment of drug therapy and the detection of any side effects;

(2)   Occupational health and safety benefits accrue from the laboratory investigations carried out when workers take up a new job and during the subsequent routine surveillances for toxicity (of CO, Pb, benzol etc).

(3)   The routine testing of blood following donation benefits both

the donor and the recipient. However, European national health authorities have different priorities in the screening of donated blood:

- All countries carry out blood grouping and screen for hepatitis;
- Syphilis screening is performed in all but the Nordic countries who consider the risk to be negligible if blood is fractionated or refrigerated for some days before transfusion;
- Transaminase levels are measured only in Austria and the Federal Republic of Germany, and malaria screening is performed for some groups in the United Kingdom;
- The routine screening for AIDS antibodies is likely to be introduced in the near future.

(4) Clinical laboratory procedures can have legal implications when, for example, they are used to establish the cause of death or to quantitate the amount of alcohol in the blood of a driver following a road traffic accident.

(5) Clinical laboratory tests are of considerable importance in epidemiological studies:

- For influenza it may be necessary to determine if vaccine strains are still useful and in agreement with epidemiological data;
- Following food poisoning the typing of bacterial strains is necessary to establish a link between affected patients and infected food;
- Epidemiological surveys are important for cost benefit analysis before major political decisions concerning health are taken.

CLINICAL LABORATORY SCIENCE - WHERE?

It is important to distinguish where the specimen is collected and where the analysis is carried out. Until recently most tests have only been carried out in public or private laboratories. However, the simplification of analytical procedures now allows patients to carry out some tests themselves. For example women may now easily perform pregnancy tests on their own urine and diabetics are able to monitor their blood glucose levels at home. In addition the ability to carry out several analyses quantitatively using test strips now enables general practitioners to make rapid diagnoses in the office. Although there are considerable advantages in being able to carry out tests rapidly at the time of patient consultation there are also problems. These relate to the failure to take adequate internal and external quality control procedures when tests are carried out by individuals with a non-scientific background.

CLINICAL LABORATORY SCIENCE - HOW?

Clinical laboratory investigations should fulfil minimum basic scientific criteria relating to sensitivity, specificity and reproducibility. Moreover reagents, apparatus and methods should be adapted to produce optimal results.

Methods are most often recommended by scientific professional societies. National authorities pay varying degrees of attention to reagents and apparatus depending on the size and political system of the country. In some instances reagents may be produced and distributed by a national health laboratory whilst in others minimum criteria are set for their registration.

The fear of manufacturers that stringent regulations could be applied to reagents just as they are to human drugs is not justified as there are fundamental differences between the two classes of products. Drugs are introduced into the human body and might be toxic, teratogenic or carcinogenic. The development of the drug therefore requires extensive animal and human studies covering many parameters. This contrasts to the development of reagents for in vitro use which need only comply with chemical products legislation. There is, however, an absolute necessity for both drugs and reagents to be of constant quality which is only achieved by the application of good manufacturing practices for production and control.

CLINICAL LABORATORY SCIENCE - HOW MUCH?

Clinical laboratory investigations currently represent about 3-5% of the health care budget and this cannot increase indefinitely. An equilibrium has therefore to be defined by political authority considering the cost-benefit balance. There are several problems in containing costs.

(1)   Prescribers are involved in the progress of medicine and are independent from the departments which carry out clinical laboratory investigations. The difference is even more acute between industrialized and developing countries. Clinicians should establish, just as for drugs, a WHO list of essential laboratory tests which applies to diagnosis and which could be periodically revised. This task is perhaps more difficult than for drugs since the results of tests depend on the reagents, the methods, the apparatus and the interpretation.

In order to limit expenses the clinical laboratory budget in France is included by the national authorities in the global budget and tests are not paid for one by one. The private laboratories are tied to a list of tests which are reimbursed by social security, but the system is not fully satisfactory as only the authorities and the trade unions representing the biologists involved meet for discussions, without the participation of the prescribers.

(2)   In the area of disease prevention, difficulties result from the variable actions taken as a result of cost-benefit evaluations. In Europe the routine testing of blood donors for AIDS, the

In Europe the routine testing of blood donors for AIDS, the serological testing of hospital workers before hepatitis immunization and the testing of pregnant women for toxoplasmosis receive different approaches from health authorities in spite of similar cost-benefit studies.

(3)   Check-up laboratory investigation for the whole population over 40 years of age is very costly and its cost-effectiveness is difficult to establish. For this reason it is highly important to select properly the parameters under investigation.

(4)   Specific tests for the prevention and detection of professional diseases are developing with the support of the appropriate enterprises.

(5)   Tests performed by individuals (pregnancy tests or blood glucose) or by practitioners with strip reagents will probably develop in the future due to their ease of use and rapidity. They are not actually supported financially by health authorities in France (except glucose tests).

8

The Clinical Laboratory in the Changing Scene of Health Care as Seen in the USA

R Nadeau

INTRODUCTION

Over the past few years, the US health care industry has undergone considerable change. This has been due to a number of economic, demographic and technological pressures. The interaction of these forces is leading to a restructuring of the practice of laboratory medicine. The role of the traditional clinical laboratory is changing, as testing moves away from the hospital to alternative testing sites such as physicians' offices. Cost containment is becoming such a key concern, that many fear the quality of health care is likely to suffer. This environment presents new challenges for NCCLS, as consensus standards become one of the key cost-effective factors in ensuring the continued quality of laboratory medicine.

ECONOMIC FACTORS

The most significant factor in the economic arena has been the enactment of prospective payment legislation in October 1983, aimed at curbing steeply rising health care costs. This measure affects all inpatient hospital services furnished under the federally funded Medicare Program, but with a few exceptions - psychiatric, rehabilitation, children's and long-term hospitals. The basis of this legislation is the 'diagnosis related group' or DRG, which can be defined as a 'clinically coherent group of diagnoses, fairly equal in resource consumption'. Under this plan a person entering a hospital is assigned to a DRG based on diagnosis, operating room procedures, age, sex and discharge status. The hospital is reimbursed a fixed fee for a given DRG, regardless of their actual expenses. Since most hospitals accept assignment, they are unable to bill the patient for non-reimbursable costs. This system has led to an extremely cost-conscious environment where hospitals are looking to minimize length of stay, increase occupancy rates and improve efficiency.

The impact of this environment on hospital clinical laboratories has been significant. More testing is being done on an outpatient or pre-admission basis; cost-ineffective procedures are being eliminated; tests for monitoring and therapy planning are increasing; purchasing practices for supplies and consumables are being reviewed; and productivity standards for clinical laboratory services are being developed. Basically, the role of the clinical laboratory is shifting from a primarily revenue-generating, service-oriented function more to that of a cost centre.

The effect of prospective payment has also been felt by commercial laboratories and group practices. Commercial laboratories are required to accept assignment and thus cannot bill the patient for any differences between their regular fees and the Medicare reimbursement rates. These laboratories are, therefore, trying to improve profitability by attempting to increase test volume for high-profit tests, improving result turnaround times and offering hospital laboratory management services. On the other hand, prospective payment has increased physicians' incentives to perform in-house testing. Since physicians need not accept assignment, their patients are responsible for all charges not covered by Medicare, as long as the tests are performed in the physician's office. For those tests that are referred to commercial laboratories, the physician only receives a token 'drawing fee'. This aspect of the new legislation has provided physicians with a means of protecting their revenues, and a significant trend towards in-house testing is becoming evident.

As a result of these developments, clinical laboratory services are being marketed much more aggressively than in the past. Hospitals are actively pursuing outpatient testing to complement their normal inpatient volume; commercial laboratories are offering numerous incentives to retain their referral business from physicians; group practices are using the availability of on-site testing as a means of attracting more patients. The net impact is, therefore, a substantial increase in outpatient testing. There is also considerable concern that this decentralization of testing could affect the quality of laboratory medicine, since the personnel performing the tests may not always be as technically competent as trained clinical laboratory technicians.

DEMOGRAPHIC FACTORS

It is possible to identify a number of demographic trends that will impact on the volume and type of testing performed:

(1) ageing of the population;
(2) rapidly increasing supply of physicians;
(3) declining office visits per capita;
(4) decline in hospital admissions.

The first two represent a strong positive influence on laboratory testing, but are counteracted to some extent by the last two. It is expected that the increase in supply of physicians will prompt the formation of more group practices, and that the number of physicians per practice will increase. This, in turn, is expected to increase the amount of testing performed in physicians' offices. Group practices will be better able to cost-justify instrument purchases, and will use in-house testing to counteract the decrease in revenues caused by declining office visits. The ageing of the population should also serve to increase the overall test volume, but will create a shift in the test mix performed.

TECHNOLOGICAL FACTORS

The environmental trends resulting from economic and demographic pressures are reinforced by significant advances in technology, which make it easier for tests to be performed in non-traditional settings such as physicians' offices, ambulatory care centres, and patients' homes. At the same time, the entire field of laboratory diagnostics is feeling the impact of technological advances in the areas of recombinant DNA, monoclonal antibodies, immune assays and computer science. New clinically significant tests are being developed, existing tests are being refined, resulting turnaround time is being decreased and patient records are being handled on a much more efficient level than in the past.

Recombinant DNA

Of all the technologies mentioned above, recombinant DNA will probably have the most significant impact on clinical laboratory medicine. Recombinant DNA research is bringing the scientist much closer to understanding the pathogenesis of important diseases (e.g. cancer, autoimmune diseases, atherosclerosis). This will throw wide open an entirely new set of diagnostic procedures which could be direct DNA procedures or tests for substances produced by identified DNA sequences. However, the more immediate impact of recombinant DNA techniques is likely to be in the improvement of existing diagnostic procedures, particularly immunoassays. Ultra-pure reagents produced by recombinant DNA technology could be used to stimulate the production of the antibody needed for immunoassays. This could make certain immunoassays more economical and hence improve their general availability. This could also improve their sensitivity and specificity and, in turn, their relative clinical utility.

Monoclonal antibodies

Monoclonal antibodies are expanding the role of immunological detection and measurement in several areas, especially infectious diseases, cancer markers and lymphocyte subtyping. Direct antigen detection tests are revolutionizing the field of infectious diseases by providing a very rapid and simple means of identifying pathogenic organisms. In the area of cancer markers, typing and subtyping tumour cell types using monoclonals may provide prognostic and therapeutic information to the physician, allowing him to select optimum therapies. Further, monoclonal antibodies, highly specific for lymphocyte surface markers, have allowed rapid progress in the understanding of the function of the immune system and its regulatory mechanisms. Overall, the use of monoclonal antibodies has opened up new areas of clinical diagnostics, and has provided an impetus towards rapid, non-instrument based testing which is easily performed outside the traditional clinical laboratory.

Computer technology

Improvements in computer technology have already impacted patient record-keeping and the handling of patient test results. It is expected that laser optical disc storage, coupled with the development of much faster and more sophisticated local area networks, will begin the movement towards a comprehensive clinical information system (i.e. the electronic patient chart). Improved computer technology will also allow much more extensive and flexible automation of the clinical laboratory, and drive a trend towards more online instruments and significantly reduced turnaround times.

In summary, this combination of the technological, economic and demographic factors is causing major changes in clinical laboratory medicine. Technological advances are opening up countless possibilities for new, clinically significant tests. At the same time, they are making it possible for tests traditionally performed in clinical laboratories to be more widely used in non-traditional settings - physicians' offices, satellite laboratories, the bedside, ambulatory care centres, and even the home. This is all taking place in an extremely cost conscious environment, which is causing clinical laboratories to re-evaluate their internal organizational needs in terms of workflow, productivity, automation, computerization and cost-effectiveness. Maintaining the quality of clinical laboratory medicine in such a changing environment is critical, and it is here that the NCCLS and consensus standards will play a key role.

THE ROLE OF THE NCCLS

In 1967, when the NCCLS was founded, the clinical diagnostics industry was experiencing unprecedented growth. Technological advances had greatly increased the power of laboratory diagnostics, and the clinical laboratory was playing a much more important role in patient care than ever before. Along with such rapid change came the urgent need for technical standards. Recognition of this need led representatives of industry, government, and professional associations to adopt the concept of voluntary consensus standards, and to found the NCCLS. Since then, the NCCLS has had a revolutionary effect on laboratory practice. Consensus standards are widely accepted by the health care industry, and the NCCLS is viewed as a primary service organization for the laboratory community.

The current changes in the US health care industry represent new challenges for NCCLS. What role will it play in ensuring that the quality of laboratory medicine does not suffer as a result of a cost-conscious environment? How will it help the industry address such issues as laboratory utilization, management and technology assessment, while still maintaining its traditional activities relating to technical standards?

Changing direction

Since the advent of prospective payment in 1983, NCCLS has devoted much time to re-examining its goals and programmes, in order to maintain a leadership role in the health care industry. 1983 represented a year of redirection for NCCLS.

Firstly, a major commitment was made to make all documents more 'reader friendly'. This effort was aimed primarily at reaching alternative testing sites (e.g. physicians' offices, group practices, ambulatory care centres) where the person performing the tests may not have the same level of technical expertise as a clinical laboratory technician. It is expected that this programme will increase the adoption of consensus standards in the non-traditional clinical laboratory, thereby ensuring a uniform level of quality in laboratory medicine.

Secondly, more emphasis was placed in the area of laboratory management. New projects were launched in critical areas such as laboratory cost containment and the application of general management tools to laboratory operations. This increased focus on the more practical needs of the laboratory, increased NCCLS acceptance in the clinical laboratory community, and therefore enhanced the use of its standards.

Thirdly, a major fort was launched to expand the NCCLS corresponding membership, as a means of increasing the impact of NCCLS standards in all areas of the medical community that deal with laboratory testing.

New projects

These efforts continued in 1984, as NCCLS followed a new direction where quality and cost-effectiveness were the key. Communications were established with professional organizations interested in ensuring the quality and cost-effectiveness of small laboratories in non-traditional settings. Various new projects were initiated in order better to serve the changing needs of the clinical laboratory:

-   A **cost-effective quality control** programme which establishes criteria for adequate control procedures, while stressing cost-effectiveness and clinical relevance;

-   A **cost accounting** programme that develops an accounting system which reflects true cost per test by factoring in all laboratory operational costs;

-   An **instrument performance evaluation** programme which will provide a protocol that enables a laboratory to evaluate an instrument's performance without extensive statistical analysis. This protocol will be particularly suited to the evaluation of new instruments, and will represent significant time and labour savings;

- A programme for the **critical evaluation of tests** which will set guidelines for determining the medical value of new tests. This will be particularly significant as new technologies such as recombinant DNA throw open a whole new set of diagnostic procedures.

Resource allocation

In keeping with this direction, a significant portion of 1985 NCCLS resources have been budgeted for expanded service in three areas:

- protecting levels of performance that are required for good clinical laboratory medicine in the face of cost pressures;

- protecting laboratories against liability because of pressures to reduce quality;

- providing laboratories with self-audit capabilities.

These various 'new direction' activities by no means alter the NCCLS commitment to providing quality technical standards for the clinical laboratory community. On the contrary, they serve to enhance the NCCLS tradition of service to the clinical laboratory by helping these laboratories adjust to the demands of a cost-conscious environment.

CONCLUSIONS

The changes initiated since the advent of prospective payment reinforce the NCCLS' position as a strong force in maintaining the quality of clinical laboratory medicine. Consensus standards are more important than ever in an environment where the role of the traditional clinical laboratory is changing, and cost containment is critical. By reaching out to the non-traditional testing sites and focusing on the changing needs of the clinical laboratory community, the use and impact of NCCLS standards will increase significantly, thus ensuring that the quality of laboratory medicine will not suffer as a result of a rapidly changing, cost-conscious environment.

Part 3

WOULD THE VALUE OF CLINICAL LABORATORY SCIENCE BE INCREASED BY FURTHER WRITTEN AND MATERIAL STANDARDS?

9

Would the Value of Clinical Laboratory Science be Increased by Further Written and Material Standards in Histology?

J Rygaard

INTRODUCTION

The task of the histopathologist is to make diagnoses on the basis of microscopic examination of tissues. Histological diagnoses, as all other laboratory results, supply the clinician with evidence for making or confirming his clinical diagnosis and his judgement about prognosis. Furthermore, when recorded in regional, nationwide or international registers, such information may be important for developments in health care and preventive medicine.

The histopathological diagnosis may influence the clinical diagnosis more than results obtained in other laboratories. However, in contrast to measurements performed in the clinical chemistry or microbiology laboratories, the results obtained by the histopathologist are influenced by the subjective nature of the procedure, particularly when it comes to semi-quantitative or attempted quantitative decisions, generally known as 'histopathological grading'. Moreover the possibility of sampling errors is greater than in other disciplines, since biopsy or other specimens may not be representative of the tissue of interest.

THE HISTOPATHOLOGIST AS A LABORATORY INSTRUMENT

How is the histopathologist prepared to perform his job, not only as a person, but also as part of the machinery in the laboratory? His basic equipment does not differ from that of others. His eyes,

---

Abbreviations used in the text

AFIP	Armed Forces Institute of Pathology
SNOMED	Standardized Nomenclature of Medicine
UICC	Union Internationale Contre le Cancer
WHO	World Health Organization

and his general experience in perception enable him to perform the complex function of pattern recognition. During medical school training and postgraduate education the histopathologist will make himself familiar with the appearance of tissues, both normal and pathological. His results are scrutinized by an experienced colleague, so that his diagnoses will conform closely to those of the team. Concordance between diagnostic criteria is obtained by the use of standard text books and reference books. Such standards, known and applied worldwide, are the UICC or WHO publications that offer the basis for international histological classification of tumours. These publications describe the biological concepts underlying diagnosis and most importantly as is the case with the WHO series, illustrate the various tumours with colour prints. Another series of generally accepted reference books is published by the AFIP. Also, the know-how of pathologists is constantly updated by reading and participating in advanced courses, so that progress in the discipline is gradually incorporated in the state of the art. Another important source of development of skills is the close collaboration with the clinician in order to adopt new concepts.

REPRODUCIBILITY IN HISTOPATHOLOGY

In spite of the training described above, and the use of the same references, it has been shown repeatedly that there may be significant differences in the evaluation of similar - or even the same - histological slides. This has been shown most clearly in studies of grading of premalignant or malignant changes, such as dysplasia/carcinoma of the uterine cervix, breast cancers, carcinomas of the larynx, or prostatic carcinomas. This has led to interesting analyses of observer variation between pathologists.

In an early study, Henriksen[1] analysed the problem of classification of dysplasia, carcinoma in situ, or carcinoma of the uterine cervix. The same sections from ten patients with one of the diagnoses were classified by 20 Danish pathologists. The diagnostic criteria used at that time differed slightly between pathologists, but when related to a given nomenclature (Vienna nomenclature), results differed widely, with four out of the ten specimens being classified as slight or severe dysplasia by individual pathologists. Another four slides had the diagnoses of either severe dysplasia or carcinoma in situ. In spite of the disagreement, one important conclusion of the study was that, with the criteria for treatment at the time, none of the patients would have been deprived of control or treated for carcinoma if this was not present.

In breast carcinoma histological grading is widely used to determine the prognosis. Delides et al.[2] assessed the reliability of the WHO grading system by asking six pathologists to grade 158 specimens independently. Five of the pathologists had been simultaneously trained in the same institution, and the sixth pathologist was one of their tutors. A high degree of concordance might therefore have been expected. However, there was agreement in the grading of only 23 out of the 158 cases, most of which were

either well or poorly differentiated tumours. The authors concluded that if the prognosis of breast carcinoma is predicted by
the WHO method, it should be restricted to the two extreme
groups, and they further conclude that it seems that there is no
need to apply the WHO grading method since these groups could be
easily distinguished by the overall impressions of the examining
pathologists.

In my own institute, a similar study of the precision of histological grading was performed by Graem et al.[3]. Their study
concerned grading of cancer of the larynx. The starting point for
the investigation was a grading system proposed by Jacobsson[4] and
modified by Lund et al.[5]. This grading system comprises not only
four tumour parameters, but also four parameters describing
tumour-host relationship. Six pathologists, all on the staff of the
institute, were asked to grade 22 biopsies with the diagnosis of
carcinoma of the larynx, the grading being based on the eight
parameters of the system. Careful statistical analysis was applied
to determine the noise components in the system. It proved that
the noise of greatest importance was created between the
pathologists in their ranking of the patients on the scale of malignancy. Furthermore, the pathologists used the individual items
differently, and certain items seemed to conform little to the scoring system. An attempt was made to minimize the last two components by statistical methods. However, neither calibration of the
pathologists, nor the omission of the deviating items improved the
precision.

This may seem to be a very sad conclusion. The basic
problem in this and similar attempts to make scoring systems in
histopathology may not be basically due to observer variation.
Some of the items may actually describe the same biological
phenomenon, the importance of which for tumour spread and therefore prognosis is not known at the present time. One area of confusion in grading systems involving tumour-host relationship is the
importance of tumour leucocytic infiltration in relation to host
defence mechanisms and prognosis. Kreider et al.[6] have recently
reviewed this problem. Their aim was to examine the hypothesis
that infiltrating leucocytes of human and experimental tumours are
components of the host immunological defence against the tumour,
and favourable for prognosis. They conclude that leucocytic infiltration includes such diverse mechanisms as tumour cell lysis,
cytostasis or stimulation of proliferation, and that the present state
of our knowledge precludes broad generalization of mechanisms.
Such studies, rather than discouraging the idea of grading, should
encourage the utmost care in selection of criteria.

Recently a study of prostatic carcinoma grading was performed by two investigators using two different grading systems[7].
Randomly selected prostatic carcinomas were regraded resulting in
intraobserver agreements of 65% and 42% in one grading system,
versus 90% and 71% with the other system. Interobserver agreements were 36% and 69% respectively for the two systems. Although the latter system appears to be better, it seems that
further elaboration and standardization in this area is necessary.

MEDICAL STATISTICS AND STANDARDIZATION

The need for uniform diagnoses, i.e. standardization in histopathology, is stressed by ongoing studies concerning certain malignant diseases such as, in Denmark, the treatment of Hodgkin's lymphomas, testicular tumours, and breast cancer. As part of these studies, small groups of pathologists have been formed to evaluate all patients in the protocols. This cannot - and should not - be done for all histopathological work, but it emphasizes the need for standardization. This same need is obvious when it comes to nationwide medical statistics. A recent publication from the Danish Cancer Registry[8] demonstrated differences between the various counties in Denmark on the basis of the relationship between the incidence rates for carcinoma, carcinoma in situ and severe dysplasia. The differences were found both for all precancerous lesions relative to invasive carcinoma, and for carcinoma in situ and severe dysplasia. On the basis of inquiries to the various pathological institutes, the authors concluded that differences in the relationship between carcinoma in situ and severe dysplasia are probably due to differences in classification between the institutes, combined with the coding practices of the Danish Cancer Registry. The authors recommended that an effort should be made to employ a common nomenclature making classification possible for the benefit of international comparability and for comparisons with previous registrations.

This problem has also become evident in recent years in that computer based filing systems have been introduced in many hospitals, some using individual computers, and others being connected to the Kommunedata pathology system, which is a joint venture of many, but not all, local authorities in Denmark. The coding system used is based on the SNOMED system, authorized in modified form by the Danish Department of Health. The system is a multiaxial, hierarchical system, logical in structure, but somewhat inflexible. However, it is extremely important that such centralized registers be standardized in order to allow international comparability. This is another important area for standardization which calls for a more refined coding system that can be broadly accepted.

STANDARDIZATION OF REAGENTS

There is a need to standardize biological reagents used in histology. The development of monoclonal antibody techniques has provided the pathologist with a range of reagents opening a totally new world to diagnosis. International groups are already deeply involved in collaborative studies of sets of monoclonals which may differentiate, at a molecular level, cells and tissues that appear identical even to the best pathologist's eye. If the general pathologist is not going to be drowned in this flood, rapid help is needed in the form of recommendations and standardizations.

CONCLUSIONS

The picture painted here of histopathology may be somewhat confusing. In spite of good training and good intentions histopathologists cannot agree on diagnoses. Nomenclature varies not only from country to country, but from county to county. Observations cannot be expressed in figures, but only in words. But maybe we could also learn the word **standardization**!

References

1. Henriksen B, (1972). Dysplasia, carcinoma in situ eller carcinoma cervicis uteri. Ugeskr Laeg, 134, 2423-2430.
2. Delides GS, Garas G, Georgouli G, Jiortziotis D, Lecca J, Liva T and Elemenoglou J, (1982). Intralaboratory variations in the grading of breast carcinoma. Arch Pathol Lab Med, 106, 126-128.
3. Graem N, Helweg-Larsen K and Keiding N, (1980). Precision of histological grading of malignancy. Acta Pathol Microbiol, Scand Section A, 88, 307-317.
4. Jakobsson PA, Eneroth CM, Killander D, Moberger G and Mårtensson B, (1973). Histological classification and grading of malignancy in carcinoma of the larynx. Acta Radiol, 12, 1-8.
5. Lund C, Sogaard H, Jorgensen K, Elbrond O, Hjelm-Hansen M and Andersen AP, (1977). Histological grading of epidermoid carcinomas in the head and neck. Dan Med Bull, 24, 162-166.
6. Kreider JW, Bartlett GL and Butkiewicz BL, (1984). Relationship of tumor leucocytic infiltration to host defense mechanisms and prognosis. Cancer Metast Rev, 3, 53-74.
7. Storm HH and Moller-Jensen O, (1985). Regional forskel i cervikale praekankroser. Et klassifikationsproblem. Ugeskr Laeg, 147, 1137-1140.
8. Svanholm H and Mygind H, (1985). Prostatic carcinoma. Reproducibility of histologic grading. Acta Pathol Microbiol Scand Section A, 93, 67-71.

10

Would the Value of Clinical Laboratory Science be Increased by Further Written and Material Standards in Cytopathology?

OAN Husain

INTRODUCTION

Good laboratory practice may be defined as the provision of an accurate, reliable, economic and effective diagnostic service within a reasonable time interval acceptable to clinician and patient. It is effected by the creation of a balanced structure of laboratory service where building, space, equipment, workforce, administration and atmosphere compound to provide a harmonious, stressless and efficient service. There is no doubt whatsoever that the use of additional written and material standards will further promote good laboratory practice in diagnostic cytology and this paper will consider the importance of standardization in achieving this objective.

THE DEVELOPMENT OF THE PRACTICE OF CYTOLOGY IN THE UNITED KINGDOM

Ten to fifteen years ago cytology moved substantially from simple screening for cervical cancer to a broadly based diagnostic service. This new and developing science lying somewhere between the practices of histopathology and haematology became more clinically orientated, coping with relatively large numbers of varied routine tests all manually processed and interpreted. The mixture of screening and pre-screening normal populations for cervical neoplasia differed widely from either the fine needle aspirations of tumours of the breast thyroid, lymph nodes, lung and liver, or the brush samples from gastrointestinal and pulmonary tracts. The latter were diagnostic and yet also sought the early lesion where prognosis was so much better.

The definition of good laboratory practice inevitably became multi-faceted and it became apparent that each aspect of a problem had to be identified and ground-rules laid down. It was necessary to develop a stratified or hierarchical labour force skilled in different practices but with each group understanding much of the ultimate interpretational target. Figure 10.1 illustrates the workflow pattern and staff activities in a relatively large cytopathology laboratory. The basic duties of the cytopathologist and cytotechnologist are outlined in Table 10.1. In addition, newer techniques and more clinical involvement make greater demands on the skills and time (Table 10.2).

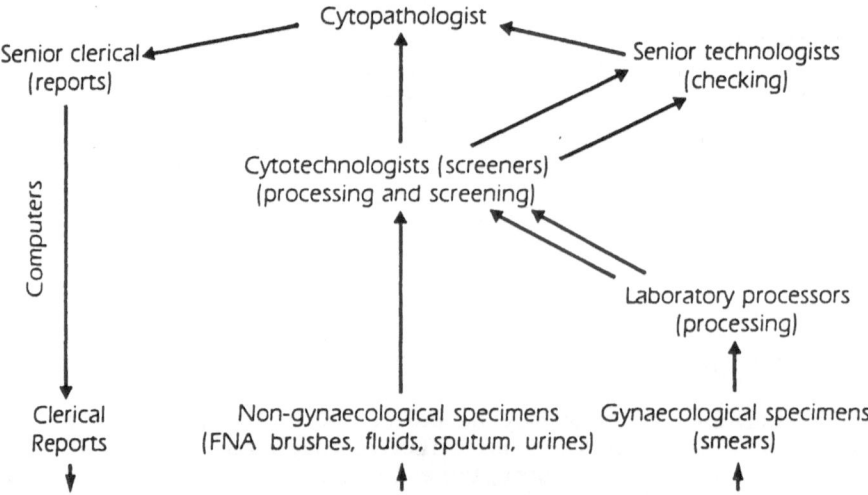

Figure 10.1 Workflow pattern in a cytology laboratory (20,000-100,000 tests per year)

Table 10.1 Basic duties of the cytopathologist and cytotechnologist

---

CYTOPATHOLOGIST

1. Establish optimum size and calibre of departmental staff, space and equipment for the service required.
2. Establish and maintain efficient and reliable work flow to provide a satisfactory service.
3. Create formal training programmes and a variety of in-service experience with seminars and case studies to achieve high quality staff.
4. Create and maintain a comprehensive, lucid and accurate laboratory technique manual in conjunction with the chief technologist.
5. Maintain high morale and good working conditions.
6. Organise and maintain quality control procedures with the chief cytotechnologist. Make periodical reports to central authority.
7. Report all abnormal smears and be closely involved in a proportion of others (10-30%).
8. Keep abreast of current advances and undertake research and development.

Table 10.1 continued

CYTOTECHNOLOGIST

1.   Identify slides and match with request forms.
2.   Comprehensively screen the whole of the smear material.
3.   Report on adequacy of smears.
4.   Report on freedom from malignancy and its precursors.
5.   Assess as an optimal test.
6.   Identify other significant findings (e.g. trichomonas, atypical metaplasia, unexplained hormonal changes, cell debris, etc.).
7.   Write a short descriptive report of abnormal findings and answer clinical queries.
8.   Receive feed-back information.
9.   Accomplish reasonable and reliable output.
10. Take part in quality control exercises.
11. Keep up-to-date with processing and screening techniques.

Table 10.2 Extra duties in cytodiagnosis for the cytopathologist and the cytotechnologist

---

On the door service - Ambulatory pathology

1.   Collection of fine needle aspiration.
2.   Skin and mucosal scrapes, and brush sampling.
3.   Intra-operation sampling and 'fast' diagnosis.
4.   Attendance at X-ray, ultrasound and CAT scan clinics for deep-seated tumour aspiration.
5.   Specimen sampling and processing.
6.   Special diagnostic techniques:
                morphometry
                cytochemistry
                immunocytochemistry
                automated scanners:
                        (static and flow cell)

Codes of practice

It is the responsibility of the professional or craft bodies such as the royal colleges, universities and technical institutes to enunciate and assess the quality of practice of both the workplace and the training and examination of the labour force. This includes the establishment of a code of practice (Table 10.3) of the duties of each type of worker in the hierarchy. The recruitment of

Table 10.3 Code of quality practice (standards laid down by professional bodies)

---

1. RECOGNITION OF LABORATORIES

Workload and variety
Space and equipment
Staff structure and content
Records and analysis
Quality control procedures

2. RECOGNITION OF PROFESSIONAL AND TECHNICAL COMPETENCE

Continual assessment

3. DUTIES AND RESPONSIBILITIES OF STAFF

Clerical
Procedural
Cytotechnological
Chief cytologist's
Cytopathologist's

Table 10.4 Origins of senior cytologists in Europe

Histopathologists	35.6%
Gynaecologists and surgeons	34.8%
Physicians and haematologists	7.6%
Anatomists	0.27%
Medical cytologists	8.85%
Non-medical graduates	12.85%
	———
	100.00%

---

cytologists from a variety of backgrounds (Table 10.4) makes the
training and examination of a cytologist difficult to standardize internationally. It is therefore necessary to have a code of practice
related to a central core of skills and knowledge married to
whatever specialist interest there may exist in any particular
country. Nowadays the use of cytochemical, immunocytochemical
and quantitative techniques in the isolated cell are becoming
paramount in the interpretation of diseases, especially in their pre-
disease states, and these skills are necessary across much of the
labour force within the cytology laboratory. It is here that a fully
competent and extensive laboratory manual must exist in each
laboratory detailing the methods and procedures required for
processing different samples and seeking different specialized en-
tities within the cell. Such manuals should be kept up-to-date and

each page of techniques should, for instance, have the date on which it was prepared in case there is a subsequent issue that updates that particular edition.

THE CYTOLOGICAL WORKLOAD OF DISTRICT GENERAL HOSPITALS IN THE UNITED KINGDOM

In order to identify and cost the demands made on the laboratory staff and to create a properly structured work pattern we analysed by time and motion study the activities of various members of the workforce in eight different types of cytopathology laboratory. Some surprising results emerged. For example, cytotechnicians basically employed for screening were also given other duties since screening could not be performed for eight hours a day due to boredom and fatigue.
A summary of the results is given below.

(1)   Average throughput per annum per district general hospital laboratory: 15,000-20,000 gynaecological smears; 2,000-2,500 non-gynaecological specimens (6,000-7,000 smears).

(2)   Trained cytotechnician output per annum: 6,000-7,000 smears, comprising either 5,000 gynaecological tests (assuming one third to require two smears), or 2,000 non-gynaecological specimens (assuming a mean of three smears per specimen).

(3)   Technicians' proportional screening time: 35% (teaching hospital); 45% (non-teaching hospital).

(4)   Number of technicians needed for average D.G.H. output: 3.4 (whole time equivalents) + 1 senior or chief technician (non-teaching hospital) 4.6 (whole time equivalents) + 1 senior + 1 chief technician (teaching hospital)

(5)   Cytopathologist output per annum:
7,000-7,500 total smears after screening by technicians (non-teaching hospital);
4,500-5,000 total smears after screening by technicians (teaching hospital).

(6)   The present workload in a D.G.H. serving a population of 250,000 equates to the work of a full-time cytopathologist in a non-teaching hospital, and probably one and a half in a teaching hospital.

Such data is not universally applicable and would probably not pertain to each and every form of laboratory or clinico-laboratory practice in each constituent country in Europe, but it does demonstrate the need for more detailed written and material standards by which to structure our work force.

QUALITY CONTROL

Internal quality control

There are several areas which can be dealt with effectively by internal quality control procedures starting with **specimen collection**. Inadequate sampling may be due to difficult or somewhat obese patients, poor sampling instruments, an unskilled collector or the spreading of the smear and fixation.   When it comes to **identification** there can be errors all along the line from the moment of sampling to the final report.   In **processing** the risks lie in sampling, fixation, stain schedules and staining instruments, where cross-contamination is a real danger resulting in false positive reports.

With **screening** the aim is to identify the smear changes as within normal limits and not to look just for the cancer cell.   The error rates of failure to detect change due to fatigue or inexperience can be measured by rechecking a series of negative cases.   This has been done in a survey conducted by Dr Yule in Manchester where he recalled over 14,000 patients with normal smears after three months (Table 10.5).   Out of the 25 cases which became positive on the second occasion 16 were found to have been negative in the initial screen, probably as a result of sampling errors, and 9 smears had been incorrectly classified initially due to screener error.

In **diagnosis and reporting**, errors can creep in when all the smears relating to the case are not present.   It is important that the number of smears made and the stains involved are fully recorded so that no-one considers the case without a full set of slides available.   Even with these precautions, diagnosis and reporting have sometimes been demonstrated to be discrepant between authorities and even by the same authority on different occasions.   **Storage and records** need to be closely controlled and 'disease indices' made so that reference can be made fairly quickly. **Histological correlation** is an important monitor of cytology though errors can equally well occur in histology when the biopsy is small.   Therefore the final arbiter is the   **clinical correlation** of these factors, which is a very salutary monitor of the final truth.

Quality control should not be mentioned without referring to laboratory safety and here very strict rules should be adhered to with regard to the use of materials and apparatus within the laboratory, where exposure to chemical and biological hazards can occur.   Safety notices should be widespread around the laboratory and incorporated in the laboratory manual.   Periodic testing of personnel with regard to these matters should be carried out.

Table 10.5 A review of the first smear after finding 25 new positive smears on re-screening 14,437 subjects 3 months after their initial screen

---

Review of first smear

	No.	Rate per 1000
Negative	16	1.11 (? sampling error)
Positive	9	0.62 (screener error)
Total ("missed" positives)	25	1.73

Calculation of error rate

	No.	Rate per 1000
Positives at first screen	143	9.91
"Missed" positives	25	1.73
True positives	168	11.64

Error rate	=	25/168	=	14.9%

With acknowledgements to Dr Yule, Christie Hospital, Manchester

External quality assessment

This may be carried out in several ways:

(a) By **inspectorates** where individuals come into the laboratory with test slides and put the cytotechnicians and senior staff through a test of interpretation. This procedure is not favoured on this side of the Atlantic;

(b) By **retrospective review systems** where the laboratory is instructed to examine the fiftn abnormal smear of the fourth month of a particular year. Such a practice has not gained favour as it is of no great interest and hardly tests the system adequately without much additional expensive peer review involvement;

(c) By **paired laboratory trials** where two laboratories exchange slides to see how close they come to agreement. When there is a disagreement it is obviously impossible to say who is correct without peer review;

(d) By **laboratory cluster circulation**. Here five or six laboratories will circulate a number of smears and then return their results to a central monitoring source so that charts can be drawn up to compare the results of the test against the originating laboratory or against a consensus.

This is a much more self-contained system and does allow for more harmonious and balanced activities where the cost is borne almost equally between participating laboratories. The results of a recent trial of such an exercise are given in Table 10.6.

Table 10.6 Percentage agreements in cytology and histology in combined external quality assessments, from a cluster of five laboratories performed in five-week cycles (From Ref. 5)

	Major categories (benign,CIN, malignant)	Minor categories (type of CIN and/or type of tumour)
Cervical cytology	87%	81%
Sputum cytology	83%	72%
Gynaecological histology	90%	91%
Respiratory histology	98%	75%
Cytology/histology/ (gynaecological)	75%	64%
Cytology/histology/ (respiratory)	91%	61%

CONCLUSIONS

The whole of this account from the basic codes of practice through internal and external quality control procedures should be defined and set up in written and material standards similar to those outlined. These have been found satisfactory and rewarding in developing and maintaining the high quality service and in fact give a high degree of job satisfaction to those involved.

FURTHER READING

1. Cocker J, Fox H and Langley FA, (1968). Consistency in the histological diagnosis of epithelial abnormalities of the cervix uteri. J Clin Pathol, 21, 67-70.
2. Barr WT, Powell DEB and Raftan JB, (1970). Cellular contamination during automatic manual staining of cytological smears. J Clin Pathol, 23, 604-607.
3. Husain OAN, Butler EB, Evans DMD, MacGregor JE and Yule R, (1974) Quality control in cervical cytology. J Clin Pathol, 27, 935-944.
4. Husain OAN, (1975). Quality control in cytological screening for cervical cancer. Tumori, 62, 303-314.
5. Husain OAN, Butler EB and Woodford FP, (1984). J Clin Pathol, 37, 993-1001.

11

Would the Value of Clinical Laboratory Science be Increased by Further Written and Material Standards in Microbiology?

AHW Wahba

INTRODUCTION

In health care, the planners, providers and consumers have four basic concerns constituting a logical sequence: efficacy, efficiency, equity and quality. Above all, the health services have to be capable of producing the desired effect in overcoming and avoiding illness, disability and death. However, owing to many constraints, a service may not always achieve its full potential. As a consequence, the effectiveness of the service - the relationship of the actual impact to the theoretical impact in an ideal setting - has to be assessed. Hence the next step consists of determining the efficiency of the service considering delivery, outcome, cost and alternatives. Once the most appropriate approach has been demonstrated, an equitable distribution of the services can be envisaged in accordance with the real needs, and not the demands, of the population. Last but not least, a high quality of the services must be ensured. In any of these four phases, standards of various kinds are involved.

When a national health care programme is planned, developed or revised, a valid laboratory support must be clearly outlined by identifying and budgeting for the necessary laboratory tests at every level of care, in such a manner that performance standards are maintained in the provision of all laboratory results. In the present paper, various factors which influence the outcome of health care and which could be improved by the availability of standards in the field of microbiology will be elaborated.

STANDARD TERMINOLOGY

Of all the laboratory disciplines, microbiology stands out as a jungle of terms. Names of microorganisms, of methods, of individual tests, of antigens and antibodies, of media, of reagents, of antibiotics, of apparatus and even diseases vary widely from one country to another and even within the same country. Laboratory personnel also enjoy a similar state of affairs, as at least 15 different categories of laboratory workers are known to exist in various parts of the world: their job descriptions are often similar, but their denominations differ.

Various international and national bodies have proposed solutions for standardizing terminology but there is still a great need for the professions, industry and administrations to agree on a common nomenclature. Within a homogeneous group of workers, some success has been achieved, but the main factor which renders agreement difficult is the multidisciplinary nature of microbiology where scientists from various backgrounds (basic sciences, medicine, veterinary medicine, hydrobiology, food science, molecular biology, agriculture and many more) are expected to work together in one and the same health care system.

STANDARDS IN MICROBIOLOGY

Source and content

The sources as well as the contents of standards could originate from a wide variety of proposals coming from individual scientists, professional societies, health authorities, non-governmental professional bodies, manufacturers and intergovernmental agencies, the ECCLS being one of them. Standards could also be developed from already existing documents but priorities should be clearly defined.

Measurement scales

In order to ensure objectivity, verifiability, uniformity and specificity, certain principles for criteria have to be laid down for any standard. Microbiology is one of the more difficult areas, as many observations and results are judged by human interpretation. Automation and computerization may partly solve the problem but at the same time more pertinent standards have to be developed.

Acceptability and consensus

When the need for a standard in microbiology is recognized, work can immediately be started when a suitable and technically competent body is identified. Apart from the main objective which is to supply reliable, accurate and precise laboratory data, other important aims such as providing the bases for valid comparisons of epidemiological investigations, health surveys, environmental monitoring and microbiological research should be kept in mind. Therefore wide-ranging consultations should be organized to obtain the views and comments of defined and potential users of every standard considered. This mechanism will ensure conditions for consensus or substantial agreement, but does not necessarily provide a unanimity on the scope, explicitness and utilization of the standard.

Transferability

Standards in microbiology, just as in other laboratory disciplines, are often developed to fit a high level of stringency. As it is well known that the level of microbiological work differs enormously in various parts of the world, the possibility of the usefulness and uselessness of certain standards must be considered right from inception. In that case, standards may often become a most welcome tool to upgrade existing health care services.

New technologies

A vast spectrum of microbiological methods has been introduced in the last few years, including visualization of an aetiological agent (special stains, phase contrast), testing for soluble antigen using specific antisera (latex tests, coagglutination, CIE, RIA, ELISA, LAL), identification of substances elaborated by microorganisms (toxins, liquid gas chromatography) and the search for substances produced by host reactions (IgM demonstration, fluorescent antibody seroagglutination).

Furthermore there are many other methods for the direct automated identification and antibiotic sensitivity determination of microorganisms which are becoming widely used. Bioluminescence, bioimpedometry and other rapid diagnostic methods, may still be in the research stage, but will soon be part of the routine laboratory workload.

All these newer technologies are in great need of standards especially since many of them will be used at a peripheral level, where highly skilled and experienced laboratory workers may not be available.

Specific areas of applicability in health care

(a)   Predictive activities such as determination of levels of immunity or susceptibility.

(b)   Diagnostic activities such as isolation and identification of microorganisms, serological and immunological tests.

(c)   Follow-up of infections such as immunoglobulin determinations.

(d)   Quality assessment schemes.

(e)   Production and control of prophylactic, diagnostic and therapeutic substances such as antigens, antibodies, sera and vaccines.

(f)   Surveillance and monitoring of water, food and environment.

(g)   Microbiological academic and applied research.

(h)   Reference materials where the standards should include criteria for selection, validation and characterization as well as specifications for production.

IMPLEMENTATION

Once standards have been accepted and their clinical relevance and usefulness agreed, a coordinated approach for their implementation should be initiated and followed up.   Microbiologists, health laboratory authorities and industry should collaborate, and an organization such as ECCLS should be instrumental both in their implementation and their development.

Effective and efficient national laboratory organization, management and resource allocation coupled with good communication at all levels in the health care system would be a major contributing factor for the generalized appropriate utilization of standards.   Reliable methods, reagents, media and instruments controlled by pertinent standards will provide the necessary timely, precise and accurate laboratory results to meet patient and community needs.

At present there are more than 500 different types of tests which are routinely carried out in more than a 100,000 health care laboratories world-wide.   In addition there are a further 500 types of analyses requested for more specific health and health-related problems.   It is therefore essential that the laboratory scientist is able to select and safely use the tools most appropriate to his needs according to defined, recognized and accepted standards.

In the present world where very versatile regions alternate with more homogeneous ones, and where different national laboratory organizations often function side by side, it becomes even more important to develop standards.   All individuals and organizations having a direct concern with the scope and provision of standards can, through a concerted effort and approach, achieve a great deal.   In Europe, ECCLS has been identifying and developing standards for which there is reasonable expectation that a consensus can be achieved.   In areas where consensus may be difficult to obtain, the pros and cons and other arguments may still be useful for any future developments.

QUALITY AND EFFICACY

In view of the present trends of rationalization of laboratory services, the replacement of certain traditionally used tests by new ones and a more systematic approach to the evaluation of all tests, assessment of efficacy is now attempted in addition to determining sensitivity, specificity and clinical value.   The numerous questions to be addressed in an evaluation of efficacy could include the following:

(1)   Does the test perform as expected?

(2)   Does the intended use of the results correspond to the

reason for requesting the test?

(3)   Does the test help in making a prophylactic, diagnostic, therapeutic, prognostic or rehabilitative decision?

(4)   Does the test eliminate the need for other procedures or simply provide non-essential supplementary information?

(5)   Does the interpretation of the test result have an impact on the final health status of the patient or the community?

Both the availability of reliable standards and the adequate functioning of quality assessment schemes ensure the sound performance of the efficacy evaluation.

The pooling of resources and expertise, being one of the main objectives of ECCLS, is particularly important in microbiology which continues to expand rapidly and still requires the validation of many of its methods.

CONCLUSIONS

(1)   National health authorities, national and international professional bodies, individual laboratories, laboratory workers and manufacturing establishments have an important role to play in proposing, developing and utilizing standards.

(2)   In Europe, where substantial information, facilities and expertise are available, ECCLS is the appropriate body for the organization, development and coordination of standardization activities.

(3)   The rapidly progressing discipline of microbiology is in great need of more standardization activities which, once implemented, will raise the level of health care service for patients and community.

REFERENCES

1.   Marchiaro G and Serra R, (1984).   Rapid methods in microbiology. Clin Chem Newsletter, 4, 50.
2.   Wahba AHW, (1978).   Some international aspects of laboratory standards.   Expert panel on structure and function of a proposed ECCLS.   Analytica. (Munich), 19, 2.
3.   Wahba AHW, (1979).   Clinical laboratory standards; the role of the health authorities. ECCLS meeting with Health Authorities. Brussels, 25th April.
4.   Wahba AHW, (1983).   The needs of clinical laboratories in Europe as seen by the Health Agencies.   ECCLS Seminar, Canterbury, 31st March - 1st April 1981.   Industry and the Clinical Laboratory.
5.   Wahba AHW,   Appropriate technology and utilization in the health laboratory. Br Med J (in press).
6.   World Health Organization, Geneva and Copenhagen. (1984). Assessment of benefits and costs of clinical laboratory testing.   Document LAB/84.5

12

Would the Value of Clinical Laboratory Science be Increased by Further Written and Material Standards in Immunology?

I Batty

INTRODUCTION

In the late '60s most immunologists involved in laboratory work related to patient care held the view that their first priority was to work towards improving the quality of immunological reagents. Commercially prepared reagents were already an essential part of laboratory immunologists' test systems, and it was believed that without standardized comparison materials, the quality of these reagents would be variable.

The main factors which determine how well a scientist controls in vitro reagents and test systems and, hence, the results produced by the laboratory, are expense, time and inclination, and it would therefore be expected that this area would be least in need of standardization. The pressures today are such that not only are the first two factors limiting but many immunological tests are becoming routine and are carried out in ever-increasing numbers, sometimes by staff who, though competent, are insufficiently aware of the basis of the tests, so that errors once introduced may go unchecked.

The lack of time and money means that few laboratories have the facilities to set up their own series of 'normal' or reference ranges, particularly for those substances which occur rarely or where the need to make the measurement is infrequent. Nevertheless, the need for such a body of reliable information to help in the interpretation of laboratory results is self-evident.

The purpose of standardization in clinical immunological laboratory work is to facilitate the exchange of reliable information for use in patient care, research and teaching. This exchange should be possible not only amongst clinicians, hospitals and laboratories in a particular country, but also across national boundaries. In spite of any impediments due to differences in legislation, standardization must be planned and carried out in such a way that the results are applicable world-wide in countries at different stages of development and with different kinds of laboratory organization.

Definition

Standard is a multi-purpose word and scientists have, indeed everybody has, the right to use it as they see fit, provided always that what is meant is clear either by context or by definition. Unless otherwise stated in clinical immunology, a standard is a comparison material. It may be for international, regional, national or inter-laboratory use.

HISTORICAL OVERVIEW

Biological standardization started at the end of last century when Ehrlich (1897) realised that if the interactions of toxins and antitoxins were to be studied in more than the most superficial way and used in a clinical context, it would be necessary to have reproducible methods of assay. He therefore produced, in 1897, his classical work on the standardization of diphtheria toxin. This, together with the work of Kraus[1], who showed that when a soluble antigen meets its homologous antiserum a visible precipitate is formed, provided the foundation for immunological standardization.

It is necessary first to consider which immunological parameters are the most useful aids to the clinician in his treatment of the patient. The WHO consultation/working group on the use and abuse of laboratory tests in clinical immunology[2] graded tests according to their usefulness in patient care:

(a)   essential for diagnosis, prognosis and monitoring;
(b)   useful but optional;
(c)   of interest for research only; and
(d)   useless in the circumstances.

Their primary goal was to define tests which would help the patients in the most cost-effective way.

The standardization of immunological reagents only got underway some 15-20 years ago when immunological reagents and test systems became commercially available on a large scale and when immunological tests were being used routinely in ever-increasing numbers. At this time, several groups of workers were concerned at the quality of laboratory results, as they found that there was no uniformity in the designation of concentrations of clinically important substances in body fluids. Two studies in particular highlighted this. In 1963 Bozsocky[3] found a 940-fold difference between the highest and the lowest concentrations of rheumatoid factor recorded by 19 expert laboratories using the Waaler-Rose technique on samples of the same specimen, and a 310-fold difference (64-20,000) was recorded amongst those using the latex technique.

The information collected by Rowe[4] and his colleagues in the second study relates to the measurement of human immunoglobulins by immunological methods in expert laboratories (Figure 12.1). It was found that the estimates of the immunoglobulin content of a sample from a single specimen varied widely.

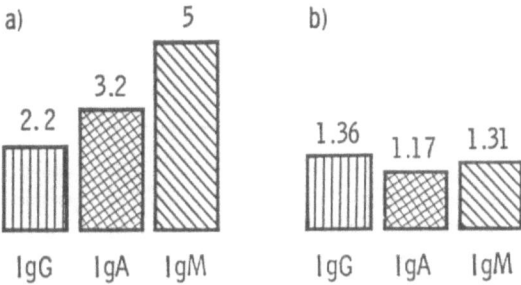

Figure 12.1   Ratios of the highest and lowest values obtained by expert laboratories measuring immunoglobulins in the same pathological serum (a) using their own antisera and antigen standards, and (b) using a common antigen standard of arbitrary unitage and different antisera

The ratios between the highest and lowest results returned were 2.2-fold for IgG, 3.2-fold for IgA and 5-fold for IgM.   The study was repeated but a common reference preparation with an arbitrary designated unitage was included in the test.   All laboratories used different antisera but recorded their results in terms of the common reference antigen, and the ratio of highest to lowest results was reduced to 1.36-fold for IgG, 1.18-fold for IgA and 1.31-fold for IgM.   This study clearly demonstrated both the need for and the value of assessing the potency of complex substances in similarly complex matrices in terms of a common standard, particularly in situations where it is often difficult to reduce the number of variables in the test system at least to any significant degree, or to define the conditions sufficiently so that the test system has a high reproducibility (precision).

IMPORTANT TEST SYSTEMS IN CLINICAL IMMUNOLOGY

Table 12.1 shows the test systems which are important to clinical immunologists.

Quantitation of immunoglobulins

The standard normally used is a large pool of human serum, preferably treated so that, when reconstituted from the lyophilized state, it is crystal-clear and can be used for all the approved methods of quantitation - radial immunodiffusion, electro-immunodiffusion, nephelometry, radio immunoassay and enzyme-linked immunoassay.   Here we are measuring a heterogeneous group of proteins and clearly there would be little advantage in using a monoclonal standard until the state of the art tells us that in these conditions it would be useful to know the sub-type or sub-class.   Then monoclonal antibodies could be very valuable. However, it is likely that in order to get all the desirable quantities, a mix of monoclonals would be needed.

Table 12.1 Important test systems in clinical immunology

Test	Condition suspected	Status of analysis
Analysis of immunoglobulins	Myeloma	essential
	Waldenstroms Macroglobulinaemia	essential
	(Heavy chain disease)	essential
	Amyloidosis	essential
	Immunoglobulin deposition disease	essential
	In the presence of biological abnormalities such as:	
	(a) an abnormal narrow band on serum protein electrophoresis	essential
	(b) presence of cryoglobulin	essential
	(c) Bence-Jones type of proteinuria	essential
	Immunoproliferative disorders	helpful
	Cold agglutinin disease	helpful
	Gaucher's disease	helpful
	Trypanosomiasis	helpful
	Bone marrow grafts	research
	Infectious diseases such as:	
	(a) Cytomegaly virus	research
	(b) Toxoplasmosis	research
	Surveys of family members of patients with monoclonal gammapathies	research
Measurement of total IgE	Hyper IgE syndrome of Buckley (rare)	essential
	Immune deficiencies and atopic families	research
Specific IgE	Allergies	not essential
	Dermographism	useful
	Severe dermatitis	useful
	High level of sensitization	useful
	Some parasitic infestations	research
Complement measurement	Genetics defects in complement	essential
	Angio oedema	essential
CH50, C3 and C4	Monitoring glomerulonephritis	helpful
	Some forms of vasculitis	helpful
	Dengue haemorrhagic fever	helpful
Immune complexes	Any clinical condition	not essential
	Monitoring rheumatoid arthritis and SLE	helpful

Table 12.1 continued

Test	Conditions suspected	Status of analysis
Autoantibodies	Systemic lupus erythematosus	ANA essential
	Mixed connective tissue disease	useful
	Chronic thyroiditis (thyroid	
	autoantibodies)	essential
	Pemphigus	essential
	Pemphigoid	essential
B and T cell	Primary immune-deficiencies	essential
determination	Secondary immune-deficiencies	useful
	Classification of	
	lymphoproliferative disorders	useful
	Selected patients	research
Lymphocyte	Evaluation of cell mediated	
response	immunity in primary immune deficiency	essential
	Secondary immune deficiency	useful
	Impairment of immune function	research

Analysis of immunoglobulins

In the analysis of immunoglobulins, the value of monoclonal antibodies for the identification of the heavy chain sub-class of
monoclonal IgG or IgA is mostly in research and here, so far as
standards are concerned, it is specificity that is the most important quality. Otherwise a standard polyclonal serum from as large
a pool as possible is the desired standard.

Total and specific IgE

Here again a good, reasonably titred polyclonal serum forms the
best standard to date.

Complement

In measuring complement as a routine procedure, there is no virtue
in using monoclonal antibody as a standard. In the research context, however, it could be useful to have standards which, being
monoclonal, react with only one component of the complex pathway.

Immune complexes

For measuring and identifying immune complexes it is necessary to have an immune complex that mirrors the one to be measured, which is itself a complex of antigen and heterogeneous antibody. Only in the research context is this a useful test. However, since Svehag and Nydegger made it known that they had two such standards validated by International Collaborative Assay 194, phials have been sent out in reply to requests.

Autoantibodies

In the detection of autoantibodies by indirect immunofluorescence the conjugate with a monoclonal class specific antibody, provided always that it has been shown to react in all expected situations by binding that class of immunoglobulin, is much to be desired. That is if it is necessary to know, with absolute certainty, the class of antibody produced as a response to the subject's own tissue, otherwise the International Standard polyclonal antisera are perfectly adequate for comparing commercially prepared or self-made conjugates. (In the author's experience, monoclonal antibodies make very good conjugates with minimal unwanted staining). However, the fashion at present is to use enzyme immunoassay.

STANDARD MATERIALS

Purity

Immunologists are primarily concerned with the activity rather than the purity of standards. It is not that it is not now possible to produce many antigens in a highly purified form, but it is an unfortunate fact that when highly purified such preparations are often lacking in stability and do not necessarily behave in the test system as they do as crude or native antigens, albumin being an example. This may give rise to non-parallelism in the dose-response curves and invalid assays. Naturally, if it is possible to prepare a pure antigen in a stable form that behaves in exactly the same way in the test system as does the native antigen, then this is a situation eminently to be desired. This being said, however, one is immediately brought into a discussion as to the criterion of purity, and some of the early confusion in the measurement of immunoglobulins and the more recent confusion in the measurement of alpha foeto protein stemmed from differences in purity of the so-called 'pure' antigens.

Of course, the position changes to some extent with the advent of monoclonal antibodies and the International Union of Immunological Societies (IUIS) Standardization Committee now has a subcommittee addressing itself to the possibility of replacing some of the standards for immunological reagents with monoclonally derived materials.

FURTHER WRITTEN AND MATERIAL STANDARDS IN IMMUNOLOGY

Criteria for material standards

Ideally a standard must:

- Have the same properties in the test system as the substance to be measured;
- Be stable;
- Be physically homogeneous;
- Be free from bacterial contamination;
- Be capable of accurate division into aliquots;
- Be freeze-dried with minimal denaturation;
- Have a uniform moisture content (1%); and
- Reconstitute completely to give a clear solution.

It is not always possible to fulfil all these requirements but every attempt should be made to do so.

Preparation of standards

This includes the essential processes in preparing a standard.

(a) Determination of need
Unless need is very clear, either because the test is difficult, or very commonly or very rarely performed but very important, no further work should be done.

(b) Writing of specifications
This is best done by an international group of workers experienced in the test system. It is possibly even better when written by one or two experts and approved by such a group.

(c) Procurement of material
Source is not important if it fulfils specifications and detailed information on all aspects of its preparation are available.
  All the standards or reference preparations IUIS is concerned with are freeze-dried according to the WHO specifications, partly for stability but mainly for the ease of transportation internationally. Although these specifications were written some years ago, they have not yet been superseded. However, such methods should always be considered critically whenever a standard for a new antigen or antibody is being prepared, or when the preparation of a standard for an antigen or antibody for use in a different situation or test system is being undertaken. It is conceivable that changes take place during freeze-drying that, without necessarily affecting potency or stability, do affect the suitability of the material for a particular purpose. An instance of this is the present international standard for immunoglobulins G, M and A which, though highly satisfactory for radial immunodiffusion, reconstitutes to give a slightly turbid solution, unsatisfactory for nephelometric measurement by automated techniques, as it gives too high a blank reading. The WHO International Reference Preparation for 6 Serum Proteins which is freon treated before freeze-drying and reconstitutes to give a crystal-clear fluid has, there-

fore, been calibrated for immunoglobulins G, M and A in terms of the first standard so that there is now a comparison material with values of G, M and A in international units which can be used in a nephelometric test.

(d) Collection of data on stability, accuracy of filling and efficacy of freeze-drying

This starts as soon as the material is in its final form. It is important that a standard shall maintain its activity without detectable loss throughout its life. But the life which you believe is reasonable varies with the rate of change of the technologies involved. One should always be prepared to scrap a standard if a significantly better one can be provided.

(e) Collaborative assay

The protocols for this are agreed, if not actually written, by experienced workers in the field with the advice of a statistician. Usually two or more candidate preparations (in the case of the serum protein standard there were five) are tested at the same time as several representative sera or preparations, using at least two methods - their own and a common recommended method agreed as the best currently available for routine work. Interestingly, several studies have shown that there may be less variation in the results obtained with one's own method than with the recommended method, largely because familiarity with a technique can compensate for its apparent deficiencies. In most cases the protocols require the establishment of dose-response curves which should run parallel over the range of the test with those of the preparations which are to be measured against it.

(f) Statistical analysis of results

This is really a part of the collaborative assay and the aim is to establish linearity and parallelism, and to confirm the suitability of the material as a standard.

(g) Acceptance as an international standard - and allocation of unitage

A submission which gives all the information under headings (a) to (f) is made to the Chief Biologicals, WHO, who arranges its consideration by the Expert Panel on Biological Standardization (EPBS) and other experts. It is accepted, or referred for further information or studies. Any queries raised must be answered satisfactorily before the preparation is formally offered to the Director General for acceptance. It can be rejected on scientific grounds. If accepted, then with the agreement of the participants in the collaborative assay, a unitage is assigned, and it becomes an International Standard or Reference preparation. Similar materials can then be calibrated against it for use as national standards and in turn laboratory workers can calibrate their own in-house standards in terms of the national standards, thus facilitating the transfer of values from place to place, and the comparison of values with established ranges of values of populations grouped by age, locality, health and disease.

Standards are thus very valuable assets resulting from a great deal of careful work, internationally and expertly validated, but before they can be used intelligently it is important to be clear on this matter of units.

UNITS

The first stage in any attempt at quantification is the definition of units by which activity is to be measured. Units in the immunological context are analogous to the international and national physical units of length and mass.

For routine work the metre is still related to the distance between two points on a wall in Paris, that is, to an international material standard just as is the international unit of human immunoglobulin G which has, by definition, the same activity as 0.8147 mg of the dry powder present in an ampoule of the international research standard for human serum immunoglobulins.

It must be remembered that there is no relationship between the unit of a specific antigen or antibody and the unit of a second antigen or antibody having a different specificity. The unit of IgE, for example, has the same activity as 0.0006562 mg of the dry powder in the international reference preparation of IgE. A unit of IgG does not precipitate the same mass of specific antibody as does one unit of IgM or one unit of ANA.

Continuity of units

Nevertheless, for any given substance the international unit is continuous and represents the same amount of activity in each succeeding standard - this is ensured by always comparing the new standard with the old in an international collaborative assay, and assigning its unitage in terms of the old standard so that the activity of one unit of material remains the same, although the weight of dry material containing this activity is likely to be different.

Immunological standards and useful reference preparations available from WHO in response to an explanatory letter to the Chief Biologicals are shown in Tables 12.2 and 12.3.

CONCLUSIONS

There are still areas where routine tests are being performed where there are no material standards. This is particularly true of the auto-antibody field, and the immunologists and rheumatologists are working together to fill the gaps, spurred on by organizers of quality assessment schemes who see the need and the value of material standards.

Laboratory immunologists believe that health care must be improved if the results are controlled by comparison with properly validated international material standards.

Table 12.2 Standards and reference preparations available for immunological use (WHO)

Preparation	Quantity/ampoule (International Units)	Year of establishment
Rheumatoid arthritis serum	100	1965
Antinuclear factor serum (homogeneous)	100	1970
Human serum immunoglobulins IgG, IgM and IgA	100	1970
Human serum immunoglobulin IgD*	100	1971
Human serum immunoglobulin IgE	11,500	1973
Alphafetoprotein, human	100,000	1975
Carcinoembryonic antigen (CEA) human	100	1975
FITC conjugated sheep anti-human Ig	100	1976
FITC conjugated sheep anti-human IgM (μ chain)	100	1978
Serum proteins (albumin, alpha 1 antitrypsin, alpha 2 immunoglobulin, C3 ceruloplasmin, transferrin)	100	1978
Human complement components C4, C5, C1q and factor B	100	1980
FITC conjugated sheep anti-human IgG (gamma chain)	100	1981
Peroxidase conjugated sheep anti-human Ig	100	1982

* British Standard

Table 12.3 Useful reference preparations available for immunological use (WHO)

Preparation	Year of establishment
Myeloma serum HL high titre of IgM ANA activity	1978
Nuclear ribonucleoprotein antibody	1983
Smooth muscle (anti-actin) antibody	1983
Mitochondrial antibody	1983

REFERENCES

1.   Kraus R, (1897). Antigen combined with antibody may give a visible precipitate. Klin Wochenschr (Wien), 10, 736 (Immune precipitation: at about the same time Ehrlich did standardization of diphtherial toxin).

FURTHER WRITTEN AND MATERIAL STANDARDS IN IMMUNOLOGY

2. Use and abuse of eight widely used diagnostic procedures in clinical immunology. (1981). Bull WHO, 59 (5), 717-728.
3. Bozsoky S, (1963). The problem of standardization in rheumatoid arthritis serology. Arthr Rheum, 6, 641.
4. Rowe DS, Anderson SG and Grab B, (1970). A research standard for human serum immunoglobulins IgG, IgA and IgM. Bull WHO, 43, 535-552.

Would the Value of Clinical Laboratory Science be Increased by Further Written and Material Standards in Haematology?

SM Lewis

INTRODUCTION

The purpose of standardization in haematology, as in all branches of laboratory medicine, is to ensure that results of quantitative assays provide clinically reliable information. They must be precise and as accurate as possible with inter-instrument and inter-laboratory harmonization. In this context standardization refers to both materials and method. It is important to ensure that the standards themselves are standardized, reliable and reproducible. To this end, ECCLS has an important role in providing the requisite specifications in written format, and possibly also in being responsible for the preparation, supply and correct use of material standards. These are major tasks and it is necessary for us first to be convinced of their usefulness in haematology. Does standardization lead to improved performance and how relevant is this to haematological practice?

IMPACT OF STANDARDIZATION

We have had the opportunity to assess the effects of standardization by observing performances of certain tests before and after the introduction of standards. A classic example is that of haemoglobinometry. By the early part of this century, several methods had been developed for measuring haemoglobin: each had its own calibration scale but none were harmonized for comparison to any other.

Thus, a 100% haemoglobin concentration was equivalent to 130 g/L by the Haldane carboxyhaemoglobin method, 170 g/L by the Sahli acid haematin method and somewhere between the two by oxyhaemoglobin.

As one might expect this situation created considerable confusion. In the 1950s, some attempts were made to overcome this confusion by recommending standard methods and by the introduction of stable standard materials, in the UK by King and in the USA by Crosby and by Sunderman and Copeland. These attempts were at best patchy and at worst ignored or unknown to the profession at large. Thus, in an international survey undertaken by the Dutch Institute for Public Health in 1962, a group of laboratories which included some of the most eminent in Europe reported the haemoglobin of the same blood to be anywhere between 110 g/L and 180 g/L. Stimulated by this situation the International Committee for Standardization in Haematology (ICSH) was formed and its first act was to set up an international expert panel on haemoglobinometry. In due course, this led to the development of an international material standard of haemoglobincyanide which was subsequently adopted by the World Health Organization. The panel also established a method standard and recommended selected routine methods based on the reference method.

An intensive campaign of education then followed, and in this ICSH received considerable assistance from sympathetic editors of journals and authors of text books. WHO published a broadsheet on the subject and manufacturers of reagents rapidly adopted the ICSH specifications in their working or secondary standards, using the WHO standard as their reference base. The results were not dramatic, and improvement was relatively slow, at least so it seemed to the impatient committee, but over the years there has been a steady improvement in haemoglobinometry in practice. This is well demonstrated by results in the National External Quality Assessment Scheme (NEQUAS) in the UK where, in regular surveys for measurement of haemoglobin, the standard deviation decreased and the coefficient of variation (CV) has been reduced to just over 1%, which is probably an irreducible minimum. A similar picture has emerged from trials in which laboratories from a number of developing countries take part in an international external quality assessment scheme. Shortly after the introduction of the standard method and reference preparation in these developing countries, there was a definite improvement in haemoglobinometry, progressively so after repeated trials during the past four years.

The success with haemoglobinometry is now being paralleled by a similar situation with the prothrombin time method for oral anticoagulant control. The variable sensitivity between different batches of brain thromboplastin and particularly between thromboplastins from different species (e.g. rabbit, human and bovine) has been the cause of misinterpretation with the resulting hazard of incorrect doses of anticoagulants being administered for therapy. The serious clinical consequence of this is obvious.

The problem is now being resolved by the fact that WHO has established a primary human brain thromboplastin reference standard and reference standards for other species, and in collaboration with ICSH and ICTH (International Committee for Thrombosis and Haemostasis) has proposed a method for expressing results of prothrombin tests as an international normalised ratio (INR). The advantage of this is that the results will be comparable in terms of the INR and therapy can be rationalized, irrespective of what thromboplastin is used for the prothrombin test. The scheme has received support from health authorities both national and international, manufacturers have been cooperating handsomely, and the proposal has been welcomed by the profession. This is a practical model for the concept of the collaboration between the three groups as envisaged by ECCLS, and it illustrates the way in which such collaboration can result in a valuable direct contribution to patient care.

THE NEED FOR FURTHER STANDARDIZATION

In other areas haematology has a less impressive record of success in its attempts to achieve standardization, but there remains a large list of what is needed. For example, in surveys of vitamin B_{12}, folate, iron and ferritin carried out by the UK NEQAS, there have been wide deviations in results, occasionally giving CVs of up to 50%. The reasons for this poor performance relate to errors in technique, failures to observe standardized methods especially with complex microbiological assay, lack of harmonization between different commercial kits and the overall lack of reference standards.

The most frequent set of tests performed in haematology is the blood count. There are now large numbers of different counters available based on different principles. They all need calibration and, if necessary, adjustment to ensure inter-instrument comparability. Whilst the individual manufacturers provide calibration materials for their instruments, there is a need for a primary material standard to control the validity of these calibrants and to ensure harmonization. These instruments have remarkable precision, and control preparations are readily available to check this. However, it is for their accuracy that standards are needed. The standards must be stable, must behave like natural blood in the counting system and must have assigned values which have been obtained by independent measurement referable to a primary metrological standard.

The European Community Bureau of Reference recently sponsored a study of monosized latex particles which appear to fulfil the requirements for a blood cell counting and sizing reference preparation. This work should be able to provide the material basis, but for it to serve its purpose adequately, there is also a need for studies of the principle of using the material as a standard in the context of the blood count, of how to apply this principle in practice, and of how to integrate it into the working laboratory with the collaboration of the instrument manufacturers. ECCLS might play a role in coordinating these diverse but complementary aspects of a most important and urgently required standardization.

Whether ECCLS should serve as the keeper of material standards or restrict itself to writing the specifications for material standards is a matter for discussion. An important function of ECCLS is to prepare written standards which relate to methodology, but its most important role is to coordinate methodology and material standards. In haemoglobinometry and the other examples described above, the material standard is the primary requirement which, for total standardization, is complemented by a standard method. Conversely, there are situations in which it is the method which is the primary standard. An example of this is Romanowsky staining of blood films. In this case the material standard is the specification for the dyes, azure B and eosin Y. The specifications for the dyes and staining method have been defined by ICSH as a tentative standard. It would be appropriate for us to adopt this as an ECCLS standard as well.

ECCLS has already produced some excellent standards on specimen collection. These include detailed specifications of specimen collection containers. However, an aspect which has not been considered in these ECCLS documents is that of laboratory test containers. Surface reaction seriously affects many haematological tests including platelet counts and coagulation factor assay. Differences in thermal conductivity between glass and plastics must also be recognized, as in time-related kinetic reactions it is important to ensure that the required temperature is reached before the kinetic measurement is undertaken. Even minor differences in the manufacturing process will affect the composition of the tubes. An ECCLS standard for specifications of test tubes, prepared by consultation between professional users and manufacturers, would be a major contribution to our common aim of reliable laboratory practice.

When defining the role of ECCLS in establishing material standards, one other policy decision is required, namely the level of standard which should be considered. Should ECCLS undertake this at the level of primary international standards similar to those of WHO and ICSH, for example, or at the level of primary national standards or secondary standards which are essentially those produced commercially for use as calibrators and comparators?

CONCLUSIONS

Although available evidence would suggest that there are considerable benefits to be gained by standardization, it is important to consider whether there may be any disadvantages. It is likely that there are none, provided that standardization is not equated with unimaginative performance of repetitive test procedures. Standardization must be dynamic and not static: both methods and materials must be continually and critically re-evaluated so that the recommendations can be added to or amended as appropriate. New techniques for the preparation and checking of standards must be assessed as soon as they become available, and these new procedures must be used if they are shown to be superior to existing procedures. It is certainly the function of ECCLS to be in the forefront of such endeavours, in collaboration with other international organizations with like interests. The work of ECCLS should be complementary to that of WHO and, in haematology, to ICSH.

14

Would the Value of Clinical Laboratory Science be Increased by Further Written and Material Standards in Clinical Chemistry?

B Leijnse

THE PRESENT SITUATION

At present quality assurance in clinical chemistry in The Netherlands appears to be satisfactory, although it is far from ideal. It
is interesting to consider whether this assertion is based only on
the belief that Dutch clinical chemists have achieved much in this
field in the past decades, or whether it can be supported by
facts. To verify the statement it is necessary to compare the
situation in the Netherlands with the proposed Standard for Quality
Assurance of the ECCLS (August 1983). In this standard the
terms **internal quality control, external quality assessment** and
quality assurance are defined as follows:

Internal quality control (IQC) is the set of procedures undertaken
by the staff of a laboratory for the continual evaluation of the
reliability of the laboratory's work and its emergent results;

External quality assessment (EQA) refers to a system of comparing, retrospectively and objectively, results from different
laboratories by means of an external agency;

Quality assurance (QA) is the whole programme of activities
mounted in laboratories, regions, countries, professional groups
and industrial companies in an attempt to improve laboratory performance generally.

Twenty eight years ago Holtz started EQA and pioneered
proficiency testing in the Netherlands. Thereafter the Dutch
Society of Clinical Chemistry founded a body organizing EQA on
the basis of the survey method. Nearly all 200 clinical chemistry
laboratories take part in this EQA, although there is no legal or
other obligation to do so. The Dutch foundation for quality assurance has not only a programme for simple external quality control but also a coupled external/internal programme assessing inaccuracy (systematic bias) and imprecision (random variation)

103

together with external evaluation of the effectiveness of the laboratories. This programme is mentioned in the proposed standard of the ECCLS.

Many laboratories in the Netherlands also take part in proficiency testing organized by industrial companies and have expensive IQC schemes. In contrast there are also laboratories which have no IQC and only participate in simple EQA. The Dutch Society of Clinical Chemistry and the CCLS (the Dutch counterpart of ECCLS) therefore continue to organize meetings and other activities in the field of QA and to stimulate laboratory participation in EQA and IQC.

In the field of QA Dutch clinical chemists enjoy a high credibility rating amongst their clinical colleagues. However, hospital administrators are generally not very interested in QA, but are preoccupied with the decreasing financial support for health care, especially in the hospitals. The credibility rating of a clinical chemist in the eyes of his hospital administrator largely depends on the statistics he can produce in relation to laboratory efficiency but not necessarily on quality assurance. This is mainly because our clinical colleagues do not identify the number of laboratory determinations they need and the accuracy and precision laboratory determinations should have. They are often remarkably vague on the clinical relevance of laboratory investigations. Occasionally a clinician even states that the level of accuracy and precision our laboratories are proud to achieve is not really necessary, and that the number of determinations is too high. However, attempts to diminish the number of requests for laboratory tests from the same clinician are often met with resistance.

Two years' experience of decreasing financial resources suggest that clinical laboratory science would benefit from an in-depth evaluation on the relevance, effectiveness and cost of clinical chemistry work. These studies should be a joint effort between clinical and laboratory staff. However, until such studies provide evidence to the contrary, it is probably fair to conclude that at present QA in clinical chemistry is in reasonably good shape, in both the Netherlands and other countries in western Europe.

THE NEED FOR FURTHER STANDARDS

As indicated above EQA in the Netherlands is based on the survey method. Essentially identical specimens are sent to participating laboratories, where they are investigated and the results are reported to the organizer. In our coupled external/internal quality control programme a statistical analysis is performed on the data submitted by the laboratories, based on analysis of 10-20 components in a lyophilized commercial control serum five times per week for eight weeks. With the aid of a computer programme reference values and standard deviations are calculated. The most important features of this programme are the detection of:

-       Systematic differences between the participating laboratories;

-    Time-related   effects that hold for a large group of participants;

-    Time-related effects in the results of individual laboratories;

-    Residual effects.

All of these effects contribute to the total variance of the submitted data.

To establish a reference value for a given component, and its standard deviation, the results from laboratories causing a significant contribution to the total variance are removed. All laboratories receive scores for their mean value as well as for their standard deviation of each serum component after comparison with the calculated reference value and its standard deviation.

The reference value is of course a consensus value, not a reference value obtained by definitive or reference methods with reference material. The calculated reference values generally appear to agree well with the values found with the best analytical methods available at the time. This only means that in the Netherlands most laboratories use methods that are reasonably specific. However, using a consensus value has drawbacks. Our laboratory, for instance, always has a very low score for total protein since our results are consistently too high. Although it would be very easy for us to adjust our calibration to bring our results within the target range, we are convinced that the reference value is incorrect and therefore refuse to do so. Active discussions on this and related topics are taking place in the Netherlands. However, true values, definitive methods, matrix effects and standard materials etc. are complicated topics, and it is not so easy to reach a consensus in this field.

Although the Dutch QA system is at present fully voluntary at the national level, the possibility that the government and health authorities will intervene and make it compulsory must be considered. In some European countries clinical chemistry laboratories are legally forced to participate in an EQA, and on site inspections may even be carried out. The inspector may bring one or more specimens with known characteristics to the laboratory and request their investigation under his supervision. However, it is unlikely that the Dutch government will intervene in this way since it knows that it is essential for the organizer of an EQA scheme to gain the confidence of the participants. In the Netherlands only the EQA organizer knows the scores of the participating laboratories. He can and does criticize laboratories with bad results and it is theoretically possible that, in a case of exceptional mismanagement, he may put the situation before the appropriate health authority.

Direct intervention of our health authorities may therefore be unlikely, but there is a real possibility that our government may become indirectly involved in QA in clinical chemistry and other types of laboratory medicine. For example, the Ministry of Economic Affairs is very active in QA in the field of trade and industry. A non-governmental body possessing the necessary competence and reliability to operate a certification system was founded last year, and later this year a body will be set up to administer a laboratory accreditation system. At the moment an ad hoc committee is busy formulating the general requirements for the technical competence of laboratories on the basis of the ISO/IEE Guide 25-1982.

The International Standards Organization (ISO) is well known in the field of trade and industry. In the ISO guide general requirements are formulated with which a laboratory must comply if it is to be recognized as technically competent. The basic requirements for the organization, i.e. quality control, instrumentation, calibration, methodology, procedures and records are stipulated and should be attainable in every good laboratory. Physical inspection of the laboratory facilities will be inevitable before accreditation.

The Good Laboratory Practice Rules (GLP) are much more detailed than the ISO guide. GLP is concerned with the organizational process and the conditions under which laboratory studies are planned, performed, monitored, recorded and reported. It was initiated by the Food and Drug Administration in the USA in 1975, due to the fact that some laboratories, despite using good methods and materials, did their work so carelessly that their results were useless. During 1979-1980 an international group of experts developed the principles of GLP for the OECD (the Organization for Economic Cooperation and Development). The OECD countries have passed or will pass legislation to control chemical substances which are potentially hazardous to human health and the environment. This legislation requires laboratory studies to be done in agreement with OECD GLP.

In the Netherlands the ISO guide will be used as the guideline for general requirements, and GLP for additional specific requirements in laboratories performing studies on toxic substances. GLP has already been introduced in the pharmaceutical industries who trade with the USA. In the next months an evaluation of the requirements based on ISO guide 25-1982 will be performed, and next year accreditation of laboratories will possibly take place on a voluntary basis. Although it is possible for a good clinical chemistry laboratory to fulfil the requirements of both the ISO Guide 25-1982 and GLP 1979-1980, most laboratories will have to make substantial efforts.

The ISO guide 25-1982 and OECD GLP are not the ideal rules for laboratory medicine, and it would be preferable for the general requirements for clinical laboratories to be formulated by experts from our own field. This problem has been discussed by a number of ECCLS experts and it was decided that rules for good clinical laboratory management and practice must be formulated by the ECCLS in order to fill the gap.

A committee will start work soon and make recommendations to the board of the ECCLS. Will the value of clinical laboratory science be increased by these new rules? The answer must be that if the technical quality of a laboratory at this moment is good, then its technical performance may not improve. However, if it is possible to have good rules for the specific features of our field such as management including the costs and relevance of the work done, an increase in efficiency is very probable.

15

Would the Value of Clinical Laboratory Science be Increased by Further Written and Material Standards in Toxicology?

SS Brown

INTRODUCTION

Toxicology used to be defined quite simply as the science of poisons, but nowadays it is concerned with the harmful effects of chemical substances upon all living creatures and their environments. Thus it is a very diverse subject which encompasses a whole spectrum of disciplines ranging from chemical and biochemical analysis, through histology, immunology, reproductive and neuropathology, to clinical, forensic, occupational, environmental and veterinary medicine. Some of these aspects have profound socio-economic implications or geo-political overtones as discussed, for instance, in the series of monographs edited by Coulston and Korte[1]. For these and other reasons many different bodies - national, international and supranational - have promulgated guidelines or criteria which have some bearing on the way in which

---

Abbreviations of the organizations referred to in the text

ACB	Association of Clinical Biochemists (UK)	IUTox	International Union of Toxicology
CEC	Commission of the European Communities	NCCLS	National Committee for Clinical Laboratory Standards (USA)
ECETOC	European Chemical Industry, Ecology and Toxicology Centre	OECD	Organization for Economic Cooperation and Development
ECO	Pan American Center for Human Ecology and Health	PAHO	Pan American Health Organization
EEC	European Economic Community	SFBC	Société Française de Biologie
HSE	Health and Safety Executive/Commission (UK)		Clinique
ILO	International Labour Organization	UNEP	United Nations Environment Programme
IUPAC	International Union of Pure and Applied Chemistry	WHO	World Health Organization
IUPhar	International Union of Pharmacology		

toxicology is approached by clinical laboratory scientists and physicians.

The information explosion of recent years precludes any attempt to offer a comprehensive review of such documents. Quite apart from the 70-odd specialty journals on the subject (Acta Pharmacologica et Toxicologica, Bulletin of Environmental Contamination and Toxicology, right through the alphabet to Veterinary and Human Toxicology and Xenobiotica), some of the major publishing houses have separate lists of titles on toxicology, and bodies such as ECO/PAHO and UNEP/WHO produce their own newsletters. There has also been an organization explosion. In the United States[2] there are at least 28 governmental and 22 non-governmental bodies with on-going interests in toxicology, and each of these almost certainly has a counterpart in one or more of the European countries. At the international level, there are several organizations (e.g. IUPhar, IUPAC, IUTox) with major commitments to some branch of toxicology, and the same is true at the supranational level (CEC, ILO and WHO). This paper will therefore present a personal and quite selective view of the impact - or potential impact - of some published criteria which bear on the practice of chemical toxicology, as it is applied to clinical medicine.

GENERAL ASPECTS

There are very few written standards, in the strict ECCLS sense, which have a direct bearing on toxicology practice. A notable exception[3] is the NCCLS standard for the development of requisition forms for therapeutic drug monitoring and/or overdose toxicology, the intention of which is to encourage clinicians to supply the laboratory with adequate background information to analytical requests. Clearly this is a laudable objective, which is tied up with the fact that toxicology is largely concerned with exogeneous substances, rather than endogenous ones. The laboratory's efforts to achieve sensitivity and specificity must be technically feasible, economically acceptable and speedy enough to meet the clinical need: each of these aspects may require reconsideration and change of methodology if the clinician in a particular case has evidence pointing to interference or interaction, or multiple dosage or overdosage. Clinicians do need to be aware that the potential for qualitative or quantitative analytical error is tremendous, even if only 10^4 out of the 1.4×10^7 known chemical compounds are relevant to clinical toxicology!

All too often, toxicology specimens prove to be unsuitable for analysis because of contamination, the use of inappropriate additives, or storage-induced artefacts. A guideline document which bears upon these important pre-analytical factors is concerned with the collection, processing and storage of specimens for biological monitoring of occupational exposures to toxic chemicals[4]. General guidelines for biological monitoring have been outlined by several supranational bodies over the years[5-9], but only now are the practical details being addressed in a way that will help the physician at the work place. Aitio[10] has also elaborated some of the OECD principles of good laboratory practice as they apply to the occupational toxicology laboratory. The report covers sources of variation of laboratory results, classifications of methods and standard materials, and assessment of quality control procedures. The report and recommendations do not yet constitute a formal publication by the WHO Regional Office for Europe, but it is hoped that they will indeed 'facilitate discussion and action' on the part of physicians and scientists who are involved in this branch of toxicology.

Before leaving the topic of occupational health monitoring, it may be noted that Aitio[10] and others[11] have indicated the importance of biological matrix reference materials, with relevant concentrations of toxicological analytes, for (internal) control of precision and (external) control of accuracy. The question has been raised as to whether ECCLS should become involved with the specification and production of material standards of this kind. The need for control materials is real enough, but the diversity of analytes and the broad range of concentrations which must be covered to suit different circumstances would make it unwise for ECCLS to venture into this area of toxicology - at least in this author's opinion.

SOME CASE STUDIES

In several European countries, authoritative compendia of 'standard' or 'standardized' methods have been put together under the aegis of professional societies which are concerned with certain aspects of analytical chemistry. Some of these compendia are devoted to, or contain sections on, toxicology. In France, for instance, a commission of the SFBC has produced recommendations on the determination of trace elements in serum by atomic absorption spectrometry[12]. In Britain, a working party of the ACB is sponsoring critical reviews on the same topic[13]. In Federal Germany, a Commission of the Deutsche Forschungsgemeinschaft has published lengthy monographs[14] on the toxicological analysis of air and of biological materials for many inorganic and organic substances and for some marker enzymes: these methods are intended primarily for monitoring occupational exposures, but they are described in sufficient detail to be useful in a wider context.

A few toxicological methods are included in a publication of the British Society for Analytical Chemistry entitled **Official, Standardised and Recommended Methods of Analysis**[15]. It is worth noticing that in British parlance, 'official and standardized methods' are those that appear in Statutory Regulations, Acts of Parliament and other official sources, e.g. the national pharmacopoeias, or have been the subject of collaborative trials, whereas 'recommended methods' are procedures that the contributor considers are likely to be useful to the analyst, in the light of his personal experience. On this basis, the chapter dealing with body fluids and faeces considers only copper, lead and mercury under the headings of official and standardized methods, whereas the listing of recommended methods includes barbiturates, bromide, cadmium, carbon monoxide, cholinesterase, chromium, copper, ethyl alcohol, iron, salicylate, and a general toxicological examination.

Interestingly, the corresponding manual in the United States, **Official Methods of Analysis**[16], devotes large sections to the analysis of residues of drugs, pesticides, trace metals and natural poisons in foods, foodstuffs and animal tissues, but clinical specimens are not considered. On the other hand, the series of **Selected Methods**[17] sponsored by the American Association for Clinical Chemistry does of course include analytes of toxicological interest, e.g. the anti-epileptic agents primidone, phenytoin and carbamazepine in serum[18]. However, 'Selected Methods do not bear the official imprimatur of the American Association. The published procedure should be superior in terms of evaluation (by a few independent referees) and thus accurately describe to the user the characteristics of the method'. This caveat is interesting because it hints at the intrinsic difficulty of validating analytical methods sufficiently well to justify formal imprimatur.

International collaborative studies offer the best way to achieve this end, but this is a difficult enough proposition in clinical chemistry[19], let alone in chemical toxicology. However, a commission of the IUPAC Clinical Chemistry Division has made good progress in harmonizing analytical methods for cadmium and nickel in body fluids[20]: studies of other trace elements are in progress. A different approach to harmonization/standardization is exemplified by the problem of the uptake of aluminium by haemodialysis patients. The picture has unfolded sufficiently well in recent years[21] to warrant CEC convening a meeting of experts who achieved consensus on the principles of monitoring exposure to aluminium[22]. These principles have been incorporated into a draft European Community Directive[23] which has been a helpful stimulus to many clinical laboratories. All too often, national or international legislation on toxicological matters is drafted or enacted too late to influence a laboratory's sampling strategy or choice of analytical methodology.

A few examples, taken from quite different fields, will illustrate the way in which some British legislation has served as a kind of standard for certain aspects of toxicology. The problem is that prescriptive limits for exposure to toxic substances, or measures of their absorption or excretion, ought to be backed up by sampling methods and analytical techniques which are scientifically sound, to the point of being beyond reproach in a court of law. Unfortunately, legislation drafting and the analytical art tend to be out of step with one another - either the former makes unreasonable demands in respect of sensitivity/specificity, or the latter exposes loopholes in the law which are open to exploitation.

The best known example of these interrelationships concerns legislation about drinking and driving, dating back to the Road Traffic Bill, 1962. This Bill empowered the courts to take account of the results of the analysis of body fluids for alcohol as evidence of fitness to drive. In consequence, a great deal of effort was put into up-dating methods of alcohol analysis and gathering new data on the blood/urine and blood/breath alcohol ratios, in anticipation of the Road Safety Act, 1967. This Act made it an offence to drive with alcohol in blood or urine above prescribed concentrations, with breath testing to be used only for the purpose of

roadside screening by the police.   It is well known that the Act
was an effective deterrent to drunken driving for several years,
but its impact clearly waned.   This was the stimulus which led, in
1976, to establishing the Blennerhasset Group for the purpose of
evaluating roadside and substantive devices for breath alcohol
analysis.   The Group's formal report on the Intoxilyser, In-
toximeter and Breathalyser instruments was published[24], and so it
came about that the 1981 amendment to the Road Traffic Act allowed that the analysis of breath could be substantive in certain
circumstances[25].   There is little doubt that this change in the law
has lessened the demands which are being made on official
laboratories for analyses of blood and urine specimens for alcohol.
        The impact of British regulations for the control of
toxic/carcinogenic substances is also instructive.   Notable
landmarks in this field over the past few decades have been the
Electric Accumulator Regulation, 1925; Chromium Plating Regulation, 1931; Patent Fuel Manufacture, 1946; Mule Spinning Regulation, 1953; and the Asbestos Regulations, 1969.   Most of these
regulations are now backed up by guidance notes, issued by the
UK Health and Safety Executive (HSE), some of which contain
quite detailed information on the quantitative requirements for
workplace monitoring.   Thus in the case of asbestos[26],
'.....occupational exposure to asbestos dust should never exceed:
for crocidolite - 0.2 fibres/mL, measured over 10 min; for other
types of asbestos - 2 fibres/mL, averaged over 4 h; short term
exposure not to exceed 12 fibres/mL over 10 min'.
        However, the principles of biological monitoring of workers
exposed to organo-phosphorus pesticides are not so easy to define:
'.......In interpreting the results of cholinesterase activity determinations, the methodology used must be considered.   Only when a
single laboratory is involved can results be compared over a
period of time........Numerous methods are available for measuring
cholinesterase activity.......all except for the titrimetric method
are accurate and sensitive.....The success of any system of surveillance depends....on the availability of adequate pre-exposure
data; on carrying out the procedure on a regular basis using
appropriate technology and suitable trained staff, with full
cooperation of employees and management....[26].   In other words,
the human factor is of prime importance here, both in the work
place and in the clinical toxicology laboratory.   In Britain, the
multiplicity of valid analytical methods for cholinesterase and
acetylcholinesterase, and the correspondingly different units for
expressing enzyme activity would make it very hard to devise a
written standard that would be generally acceptable.
        Laboratory investigations assessing environmental or occupa-
tional exposure to inorganic lead have received much publicity in
recent years[8,27].   A whole battery of tests is available in addition
to estimates of blood lead concentrations;   inhibition of δ-
aminolaevulinic acid (ALA) dehydratase; rise in blood porphyrin;
inhibition of red cell ATPase;   increased urinary ALA and
coproporphyrin; and decreased blood haemoglobin.   There seem to
be national differences between the European countries in the ways
in which these tests are ranked for usefulness, depending on his-
toric practice and current legislation.   In Britain, as already indi-

cated, the law on occupational exposure to lead dates back to 1925, but the latest Code of Practice[28] relates to the Control of Lead at Work Regulations, 1980. The Code in question requires that at least once a year the medical assessment should include the measurement of workers' blood lead concentrations. The action to be taken then depends upon the lead values found, with four categories being distinguished:

Category A (<40 μg/dL)	represents at its upper limit the upper level of absorption likely to be found in the population not occupationally exposed to lead;
Category B (40-59 μg/dL)	indicates that lead is being absorbed due to occupational exposure to lead. For employees in this category other suitable biological tests may be carried out as an alternative, provided that blood lead measurement is carried out at least once every 12 months. Suitable biological tests include measurement of erythrocyte protoporphrins, aminolaevulinic acid dehydratase, urinary coproporphyrins and aminolaevulinic acid;
Category C (60-79 μg/dL)	represents the level at which the employee comes under direct medical surveillance in that a clinical assessment and any other relevant biological tests will be carried out;
Category D (>80 μg/dL)	represents the level above which the employment medical adviser/appointed doctor will certify the employee as unfit for work which exposes him to lead.

Clearly, these requirements have important implications for toxicology laboratories in terms both of the workload and of the repertoire of tests. It is noteworthy that the EEC Directive on Inorganic Lead, to be implemented in 1986, will include the option of three tests in addition to blood lead - δ-aminolaevulinic acid in urine, zinc protoporphyrin in blood, and δ-aminolaevulinic acid dehydratase in blood - but this directive is not likely to lead to any major change in the current approach to biological monitoring in Britain.

Finally, it is worth commenting briefly on the recent impact of an old toxicological hazard on the clinical laboratory, namely the classical fixative, formaldehyde. There have been lively debates in the past few years about the risks of short- or long-term exposure to formaldehyde vapour, with conflicting opinions as to its teratogenic, mutagenic and carcinogenic potentials. Most review articles[29,30] conclude that there is no evidence to suggest that formaldehyde is carcinogenic in humans who are chronically exposed to modest concentrations in ambient air during a working lifetime. The recommended limits in the UK are for a time-weighted average (TWA) exposure of 2 ppm for either 8 h or 10 min exposures. This means, in practice, that average exposure levels will have to be below 2 ppm for most of the working day if the 10 min TWA is not to be exceeded. Unfortunately it is not easy to make meaningful measurements of formaldehyde in air.

Experiments relating to clinical laboratories[31] show a negative effect of xylene and ethanol on the measurement of formaldehyde by a colorimetric method. Personal monitors and exposure tubes based on this method may be satisfactory in the industrial sphere, but there is so much potential interference in the histopathology laboratory as to make the results meaningless. There are chromatographic methods of measuring formaldehyde but they are time-consuming and expensive and it seems that there is still a lot of work to be done in this field. Currently, the effects on the human nose and eyes give prompt notice of raised atmospheric levels! The moral is that it is highly desirable to employ effective means of containment and practical methods for reducing exposure to formaldehyde in pathology laboratories[32].

CONCLUDING REMARKS

The main points which emerge from this short review can be summarized as follows:

-   Toxicology is a very diverse subject and there are many professional, industrial, governmental, international and supranational organizations with active interests in its various branches.

-   Some of these bodies have promulgated documents which are tantamount to standards for the clinical toxicology laboratory, especially in the fields of biological monitoring for environmental and occupational hazards.

-   The documents of this kind which have had the most useful impact are those which have been drawn up jointly by governmental and professional groups, with a mutual awareness of each other's problems.

In the context of this seminar, the question which must be answered concerns the role which ECCLS might play in producing relevant toxicology standards. Standard materials should be discounted because of the technical difficulties which have been outlined, and for commercial considerations which are self-evident. Is there, then, a genuine need for written ECCLS standards in clinical laboratory toxicology? At this stage, the answer ought to be 'No', for several reasons:

-   So far as chemical toxicology is concerned, analytical work is carried out not only in hospital laboratories but also in different kinds of academic and commercial establishments - institutes of public health, occupational hygiene, forensic medicine and pharmacology - not all of which can really be regarded as clinical laboratories.

CLINICAL LABORATORY SCIENCE IN HEALTH CARE

- Because of the diversity of the subject and its practitioners, external quality assessment in toxicology is in its infancy. Strong efforts are required in this direction, in order to provide factual data on current levels of performance. This corpus of information is a prerequisite for the choice and design of written standards.

- It is hard to identify topics of truly international interest and importance which are not already the subject of authoritative guidelines or criteria. Without doubt, many other topics remain to be tackled, but they tend to reflect local or national problems which would not be appropriate to consider within the framework of ECCLS.

REFERENCES

1. Coulston F and Korte F (eds). Environmental Quality and Safety: Chemistry, Toxicology and Technology. Vol. 1 (1972), Vol. 2 (1973), Vol. 3 (1974), et seq. (Stuttgart: Georg Thieme)

2. Wexler P, (1982). Information Resources in Toxicology. pp. 129-146 (New York: Elsevier/North-Holland).

3. College of American Pathologists, (1983). Standards, Reference Materials and Methods; a Practical Guide for the Medical Laboratory. (Skokie: College of American Pathologists).

4. Aitio A and Järvisalo J, (1984). Collection, processing and storage of specimens for biological monitoring of occupational exposure to toxic chemicals. Pure Appl Chem, 56, 549-566.

5. World Health Organization. (1973). Environmental and Health Monitoring in Occupational Health (Technical Report 535). (Geneva: World Health Organization).

6. World Health Organization, (1980). Recommended Health-Based Limits in Occupational Exposure to Heavy Metals (Technical Report Series, 647).(Geneva: World Health Organization).

7. World Health Organization, (1981). Health Effects of Combined Exposures in the Work Environment (Technical Report 662). (Geneva: World Health Organization).

8. Commission of the European Communities, Industrial Health and Safety. (1983). Human Biological Monitoring of Industrial Chemicals Allesio L, Berlin A, Roi R et al. (eds). pp. 105-132. (Luxembourg: Office for Official Publications of the European Communities).

9. Commission of the European Communities, Occupational Health Guidelines for Chemical Risk. (1983). (Activities of the ECDIN Project in Relation to Preventive Medicine). (Luxembourg: Office for Official Publications of the European Communities).

10. Aitio A, (1981). Quality Control in the Occupational Toxicology Laboratory (European Cooperation on Environmental Health Aspects of the Control of Chemicals - Interim Document 4). (Copenhagen: World Health Organization).

11. Brown SS, (1984). Scope and limitations of trace metal analysis. Recent Adv Occup Health, 2, 107-116.

12. Favier A, Arnaud J, Bellander J et al. (1984). Recommandations pour la mésure de la concentration du cuivre serique par spectrometrie d'absorption atomique en flamme (Comité Scientifique: Section de Standardisation, Commission Oligo-Elements). L'Inform Sci Bio, 10, 70-78.

WRITTEN AND MATERIAL STANDARDS IN TOXICOLOGY

13.   Fell GS, (1984).   Lead toxicity: problems of definition and laboratory evaluation. Ann Clin Biochem, 21, 453-460.

14.   Henschler D, (Ed). Analytische Methoden zur Prufung Gesundheits-schadlicher Arbeitsstoffe: Analysen in Biologischem Material.   Band 1 (1976), Band 2 (1978). (Weinheim: Verlag Chemie).   (See also Deutsche Forschungsgemeinschaft, Klinisch-Toxicologische Analytik (1983). (Weinheim: Verlag Chemie).

15.   Hanson NW, (ed). (1983). Official Standardised and Recommended Methods of Analysis. (London: The Society for Analytical Chemistry).

16.   Horwitz W, (1980). Official Methods of Analysis of the Association of Official Analytical Chemists, 13th edition et seq. (Washington: Association of Official Analytical Chemists).

17.   Cooper GR, (ed). (1983). Selected Methods of Clinical Chemistry, Vol. 10. (New York: Raven Press).

18.   Gerson B, Bell F, Chan S, (1984).   Proposed selected method: antiepileptic agents - primidone, phenytoin and carbamazepine by reversed phase liquid chromatography. Clin Chem, 30, 105-108.

19.   Brown SS, Healy MJR and Kearns M, (1981).   Report on the inter-laboratory trial of the reference method for determination of calcium in serum. J Clin Chem Clin Biochem, 19, 395-426.

20.   Sunderman,   FW Jr, Brown SS, Stoeppler M and Tonks DB, (1982). Inter-laboratory Evaluations of Nickel and Cadmium Analyses. In Body Fluids in Collaborative Interlaboratory Studies in Chemical Analysis (Egan H and West TS eds). pp. 25-35. (Oxford: Pergamon Press).

21.   Alfrey AC, (1983). Aluminum. Adv Clin Chem, 23, 69-91.

22.   Savory J and Berlin A, (1982).   International workshop on the role of biological monitoring in the prevention of aluminium toxicity in man: 'aluminium analysis in biological fluids' (Luxembourg, 5-7 July 1982), Memorandum on the Summary and Conclusions. J Clin Chem Clin Biochem, 20, 837-839.

23.   Official Journal of the European Communities: Proposal for a Council Directive Relating to the Protection of Dialysis Patients by Minimising the Exposure to Aluminium: No. C202. (29 June 1983).

24.   Emerson VJ, Holleyhead R, Isaacs MDJ et al. (1980). The Measurement of Breath Alcohol: the Laboratory Evaluation of Substantive Breath Test Equipment and the Report of an Operational Police Trial. Harrogate, The Forensic Science Society.

25.   Halnan P and Spencer J, (1983).   Wilkinson's Road Traffic Offences. 1st Suppl, 11th Edn. pp. 265-304. (London: Oyez Longman).

26.   Health and Safety Executive. (1980).   Guidance Note   (Medical Series 13); Asbestos (Medical Series 17); Biological Monitoring of Workers Exposed to Organo-Phosphorus Pesticides. (London: HMSO).

27.   United Nations Environment Programme/World Health Organization. (1977). Environmental Health Criteria: Lead.   (Geneva: WHO).

28.   Health and Safety Commission. (1980).   Control of Lead at Work: Approved Code of Practice. (London: HMSO).

29.   Health and Safety Executive. Fielder RJ, Sorrie GS et al. (eds)   Toxicity Report 2: Formaldehyde. (London: HMSO).

30.   European Chemical Industry Ecology and Toxicology Centre. (1982).   ECETOC Technical Report No.6 - Formaldehyde Toxicology: Up-Dating of ECETOC Technical Reports 1/2. (Brussels: European Chemical Industry Ecology and Toxicology Centre).

31.   Lee CW, Fung YS and Fung KW. (1982).   Determination of formaldehyde vapour in the atmospheres of clinical laboratories using chromotropic acid. Analyst, 107, 30-34.

32.   Clark RP, (1983). Formaldehyde in pathology departments. J Clin Pathol, 36, 839-846.

Note added in proof

Updated versions of several official British documents have been published. Ref.23   Official Journal of the European Communities: Amended proposal for a Council Directive relating to the protection of dialysis patients by minimising the exposure to aluminium: No. c150/6-C150/15. (20 June 1985). Ref.26 Health and Safety Executive. (1985). Guidance Note, Medical Series 17; Biological Monitoring of Workers Exposed to Carbamate and Organo-phosphorous Pesticides. (London: Her Majesty's Stationery Office). Ref.28 Health and Safety Commission. (1985). Control of Lead at Work: Approved Code of Practice: (London: Her Majesty's Stationery Office).

Part IV

FUTURE ECCLS INVOLVEMENT

16

Future ECCLS Involvement as Seen by Industry

G Kokholm

This paper deals with five topics which should be considered important in future ECCLS work.

1. SUGGESTED MODIFICATIONS OF PRESENT WORK TO IMPROVE FUTURE STANDARDS

(a) After a draft standard has been circulated ECCLS calls for comments on the proposed standard. In practice the same comments are often received from two or more people. The reason seems to be that a draft sent to a national organization is then sent out to several members who add comments to those of their organization. The organization then answers the ECCLS with replies based on these comments, but ECCLS also receives the comments from all the members. This gives the ECCLS committee an enormous amount of work, as every single comment has to be seriously considered and action taken.

Some type of reorganization for handling comments from within the national organization would be a great help to the committees, and would allow them to reply faster and in greater detail, resulting in a faster revision of the draft standard.

(b) It is an ECCLS rule that all replies from a committee to the commenting parties should go through the central office.

Abbreviations of organizations referred to in the text

FDA   Food and Drug Administration (USA)
IFCC   International Federation of Clinical Chemistry
NCCLS National Committee for Clinical Laboratory Standards (USA)

Normally the replies are sent out at the same time as the revised draft is sent out for comments or for voting. This may result in a negative reaction (more comments or a vote against) if the action of the committee does not cover the viewpoints of the commenting parties. It is likely that a lot of repeated comments or votes against a standard could be eliminated if the committee corresponded with the commenting parties directly, and before the revised drafts were circulated. The committee work would, of course, be increased, but if the above recommendation regarding national organizations and their comments could be implemented, the total work might even be decreased and the cost reduced.

(c) Several comments have been received complaining that a draft standard does not make reference to corresponding standards already available from other organizations. It would be preferable for all draft standards to make appropriate references and to discuss the reasons why the ECCLS should be producing its own.

2. STANDARDS FOR PERFORMING QUALITY CONTROL SURVEYS

It was very pleasing to receive the second draft standard for 'External Quality Assessment in Haematology', and it is important that similar standards be produced in other areas. In the blood gas field several surveys have been performed on a national basis, by different societies using different methods giving different estimates of the quality level. Their conclusions are confusing and show a lack of know-how regarding the real performance of the analysers. A lack of cooperation with industry may be one of the reasons for the poor results.

It is appropriate to call for further standards written in detail for each analyte or each group of corresponding analytes. The excellent cooperation between the profession and industry within the ECCLS Subcommittee on Standard for Blood Gas Analysers suggests that such standards can be produced and have a real chance of acceptance. If full advantage is not taken of facilities to achieve such standards, local standards may be produced differing in method, and of little help in the estimation of the quality of the patient results.

3. MORE INTENSE COOPERATION WITH OTHER ORGANIZATIONS

Despite personal involvement in organizations such as IFCC and NCCLS, and health agencies such as the FDA, I am often uncertain as to who is doing what in which organization, and what standard work is going on. It would be desirable for ECCLS to set up a committee including members of the

IFCC whose sole task would be to produce files containing names, organizations and their activities. Perhaps cooperation between the ECCLS Central Office and the IFCC Technical Secretariat, adding staff-power to these two excellent offices, could solve the problem. It is likely that much time could be saved by having such an 'activity/person data-bank' from which information could be obtained.

This would automatically result in a closer cooperation between different organizations and provide improved standards with less effort.

4.   HOW TO TACKLE THE PATENT DILEMMA

In production of standards in which we recommend methods and materials we cannot avoid some of our recommendations being covered by patents. ECCLS has not yet considered how to deal with this dilemma. IFCC has recognized the problem, and has set up a working group to produce guidelines to help its expert panels (called committees within the ECCLS). It would be desirable for ECCLS to work closely with the IFCC group to produce common guidelines.

5.   CONSIDERATIONS ABOUT THE CHANGING WORLD

In the future we will see several analyses removed from the traditional clinical chemistry department, and a possible period of conflict between the clinical chemist and the new staff carrying out the analyses. Blood gas equipment has for several years been an example of instrumentation used in centralized or decentralized situations. In our experience the best way to organize decentralization is simply by the cooperation of all parties concerned.

Analysers such as blood gas analysers can easily be placed in intensive care units etc. and work according to expectations, provided the clinical chemistry department is involved during the purchasing process and the supervision of the instrument including quality control and daily maintenance. Unfortunately some clinical chemists still feel that the analysis belongs to them in their own departments. However in the years to come this attitude will hopefully no longer exist.

Clinical laboratory science in future may well involve:

- Mass-production of analyses where time is not a major factor;

- Analyses of a special or complicated nature;

- The coordination of decentralized analyses performed within or outside the hospital (training, supervising, quality control, reference values); and

- Research on present and future technologies, in order to improve health standards and decrease costs.

The role of ECCLS will be to adjust present standards and produce new ones for this new situation. Furthermore industry must be ready to develop new types of analyser as decentralization requires fool-proof instruments at a cost corresponding to the new market place.

CONCLUSION

Hopefully this paper has demonstrated that in the future ECCLS will still be needed, and will be involved in several new areas as long as it is able to adjust itself to the world around.

17

Future ECCLS Involvement as Seen by Health Agencies

DH Calam

ECCLS has members from 15 countries each with a different health care system. Each system has evolved from specific national requirements which have been expressed through political decisions leading to different types of funding and more or less centralization. Thus all governments play a role as a health agency. Whatever the system, there are now recognized to be gaps between the health care delivered to the population and their wants or perceived needs, as well as between those and what is in principle possible with unlimited resources. In examining the role of ECCLS, this paper starts by summarizing some aspects of health care and looks at some features desirable in the functioning of a health care system from a health agency viewpoint, and their implications for clinical laboratory science. It then considers the characteristics and directions of ECCLS and finally suggests some future activities.

A health care system is extremely complex and its total cost is very high. Laboratory costs are estimated as 3-5% of the total but the combined US and European market for in vitro diagnostics alone was more than $5000 million in 1983, of which the largest individual disciplinary demand, from clinical chemistry, was more than $1800 million. Large though these figures are, they form only a small part of the total: the health care system in the UK, a relatively low spending country, costs 4-5 times this, representing an estimate for 1985 of $400 per head of population. For comparison, expenditure per person in Japan is about the same, in the Federal Republic of Germany and France about double, and in the USA nearly four times this level. The resources needed to meet demand have escalated. In Switzerland, in the period 1960-1980 the proportion of GNP spent on health care doubled, with a ten-fold increase in costs. In the UK over 25 years, the rate of hospital admissions and out-patient attendances increased by a maximum 2% per year, but requests for laboratory tests increased during the same period by 10% per year.

A number of factors have produced these increasing costs and demands. They include older populations with the increases in more specialization and more practitioners, the levying of fees for service, greater expectations of health by the population, and less individual financing of consultations and treatment because of central funding or insurance-based schemes. It should be noted that features of many health care systems are that there are no direct implications to the physician or patient of the true costs involved, and no rewards for exercising cost-effectiveness.

A government might be expected to look for effectiveness, efficiency and economy in a health care system. In the clinical laboratory these aims can be fulfilled by appropriate steps. Effectiveness depends on reliable equipment and the provision of reliable and valid results. These in turn can permit economies by reducing waste (avoidance of unreliable results which lead to further testing), and by reducing the laboratory costs and, especially, the hotel costs of in-patients and long-term costs. However, efficiency requires the provision of adequate and available resources, locally and not at some distance, so that response to requests for tests can be rapid. This also imposes a need for local expertise.

In trying to achieve these ends, ECCLS was formed to play an international, specifically European role, with a tripartite membership of health agencies, professional societies and industry. Its aims include development of standards by voluntary consensus, avoiding duplication of effort, and coordinating activities at regional level with marketing and cost advantages to manufacturers. In its work, ECCLS is able to draw on a wider range of expertise than may be available in a single country. It can take a politically neutral view and can work to prevent premature, ill-informed or technically incorrect decisions. Its main achievements to date have been the establishment of a forum in which the three constituent groups can communicate, not least through seminars on topics of mutual interest, and the preparation of several standards.

In considering the place of ECCLS, comparison with another body producing mandatory standards at a European level is illuminating. The European Pharmacopoeia Commission is an international body with, at present, 17 countries as members under the auspices of the Council of Europe. The commission consists of national delegations, representing their governments, who in turn are drawn from national authorities. The preponderant representation is from health agencies, with reduced roles for professional societies and industry. Although this body prepares mandatory standards, it has been unable to reach agreement about labelling requirements for pharmaceutical products and relies instead on a combination of national regulations, international agreements and a statement of necessary information to be provided in certain cases. Against this background, the controversy about the ECCLS labelling standard, which was finally voted through in all three categories of membership, was unnecessary - that the ambitious attempt by ECCLS to achieve consensus on such an important matter succeeded is a matter for optimism.

As ECCLS has become established, more working groups have been formed to prepare standards. Although this process was slower than expected in the first few years, the problems of assembling groups and drafting documents for comment and revision were probably underestimated at the outset. Now, however, a number of documents covering haematology, clinical chemistry and microbiology are in preparation. The four standing action committees for instrumentation, analyses, good laboratory practice and reference materials have no less than 17 subcommittees at work, each of which will produce at least one draft standard, and the disciplines being included continue to increase in number. A common feature of all this activity are the unwritten goals of increased effectiveness, efficiency and economy.

Nevertheless, developments in health care do not wait for standards to be written and trends must be anticipated. Some are mentioned in other contributions to this seminar, but a number can be pinpointed. Applications of development in genetic engineering with increasing use of monoclonal antibodies and DNA probes will take place. Environmental pressures will hasten the search for non-radioactive methods of immunoassay as the amount of immunological screening and testing grows. New tests and wider testing for infectious diseases and cancer can be expected. Trends towards patient self-testing and testing in the doctor's office are apparent. As methods become more reliable, the latter trend will accelerate because of the advantages it offers in a rural context, in avoiding out- or in-patient attendance at hospital, and in prompt diagnosis and instigation of treatment.

These trends pose challenges for ECCLS to act as a technical organization, to anticipate change rather than to follow it, and to increase its role and standing. Areas in which further efforts could be directed include method assessment, standards to cover technological developments and procedures and methods for preventive screening. The range of disciplines should be extended to ensure that all disciplines involved in clinical laboratory work are adequately helped in their activities. There is a great need for information to be disseminated in the form of guidelines and reports as well as traditional publications from professional societies and literature from industry. The availability of information and its accessibility to laboratory staff and all interested parties, including administrators and policy makers, pose problems of publicity.

Finally, but not least, the whole process of implementation of standards produced by ECCLS is at an early stage of development. Voluntary consensus agreement about a standard carries with it the implication that those voting in favour have a commitment to implement the standard as far as it concerns them. More is required on the part of all members if ECCLS standards are to have any meaning: the recognition from health agencies that a document might dispense with the need for legislation, from industry that implementation might carry commercial advantages, from professional societies that acceptance of standards will facilitate their activities, and from all three groups that there are gains from standardization in terms of more efficient and economic health care.

The views expressed here are personal and not necessarily those of NIBSC (National Institute for Biological Standards and Control) or of the ECCLS Executive or Board.

18

Future ECCLS Involvement as Seen by Professional Societies

M Hjelm

The questions raised at this seminar are whether health is improved by the use of standards in clinical laboratory science and, if so, what role ECCLS could and should play in order to encourage the use of written and material standards. This paper will try first to answer this rhetorical question from a general point of view, and then to point to areas where a future involvement of ECCLS would be of importance.

HEALTH IN SOCIETY

It is the task of the clinical laboratory sciences to provide biomedical information of relevance to the maintenance and improvement of health in society. This duty is traditionally conducted by carrying out investigations used for the diagnosis and monitoring of disorders in the way that they are classified at present, i.e. by characterizing non-health and, equally importantly, by helping to widen the knowledge of health.

Health can at present best be defined by the absence of non-health. It is conceptually very similar to the accuracy of a method being measured by its degree of inaccuracy. However, even vigorous attempts to rule out non-health do not prove health. This is analogous to the fact that the elimination of what are believed to be major systematic errors does not guarantee the accuracy of an analytical procedure. Nevertheless, the description of non-health is crucial for our understanding of health, and the state of health in an individual or a group of people.

A simple model for illustrating the relationship between health and non-health and factors causing non-health is shown in Figure 18.1. There is a gradual transition from a state of health to non-health, caused by (1) exposure to environmental factors or by hereditary factors, (2) acute disorders and (3) chronic disorders. Environmental and hereditary factors might not initially be experienced as causes of non-health but their effects might still be measurable by some methods. Examples in this context are (in the

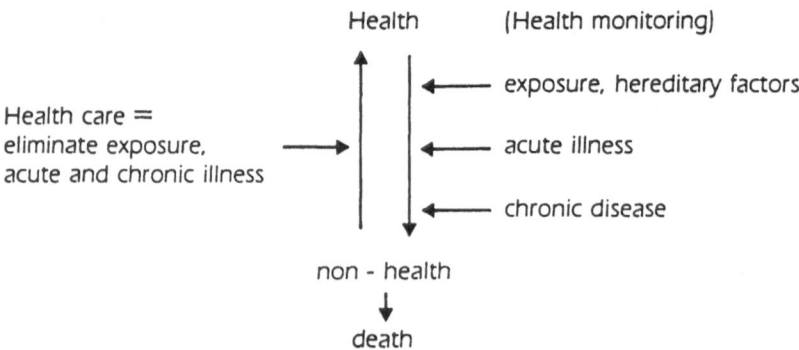

Figure 18.1   Relationship between health, non-health and death

individual)   increased   plasma   phenylalanine   in   neonatal
phenylketonuria and decreased lung function tests by exposure to
asbestos.   It is the task of health care to reverse this process by
eliminating exposure, curing acute illness and making chronic disorders less pronounced.   Only the real DNA fanatic believes that
the final step of non-health, i.e. death, can be reversed.

Other ways of characterizing non-health may be **subject
oriented** where clinical investigations are used for the diagnosis
(e.g. of appendicitis) or in the identification of a high risk subject
(e.g. a subject with an increased blood pressure), or **population
oriented**, i.e. statistical, generating figures for morbidity and mor-
tality in the general population or in subpopulations.   Obviously
the accuracy and interpretation of population statistics depend on
the accuracy of the subject oriented information about non-health.

Generating quantitative information about non-health might
involve several types of methods e.g.   the sociological,   the
epidemiological and the biomedical.   For an optimal outcome it is
required that all methods involved produce comparable results that
should be biologically relevant.   It makes sense neither to make
random samples of all men belonging to a particular age group in
two locations and to try to establish differences in, for example,
exposure to lead, if the analytical procedures for lead do not give
comparable results, nor to estimate the effect of a particular drug
in two different hospitals if the patient material is not well characterized clinically and matched for age distribution.

Achieving comparability and accuracy of results always involves some degree of standardization.   Thus the maintenance and
improvement of health should profit from the use of written and
material standards for methodology, including those used in clinical
laboratory sciences.

WHAT UNIQUE FUTURE CONTRIBUTIONS COULD BE MADE BY ECCLS?

The establishment of quality requirements with regard to accuracy and comparability of results

The professional societies in collaboration with their clinical colleagues still have the important task of establishing reasonably
simplistic rules for establishing quality tolerance limits for investigations, such that they have an optimal impact on improving
health. However, there is usually a price to pay for quality, and
whatever quality requirements are defined from an academic point
of view, such requirements have to be costed and balanced against
the money supply made available by our health authorities. There
are also reasons to believe that industry would be interested in
having its customers' demands better specified, not only to achieve
more streamlined and hopefully cheaper production, but also to be
in a position to judge what future requirements would need industrial research and development.

An interesting outcome of such a development could be that
present general indicators of methodology performance in clinical
laboratory sciences that have stayed unchanged for almost a
decade, will move again. The point is perhaps best illustrated by
an example compiled from the Wellcome Quality Control Programmes
(Figures 18.2 and 18.3).

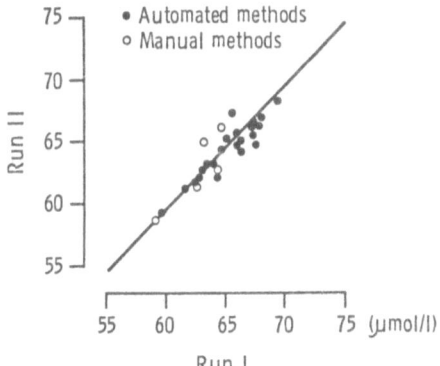

Figure 18.2 Serum bilirubin; correlation between method means (μmol/L)

Figure 18.2 plots the between-method variation for bilirubin
in bovine serum, assayed with five month intervals between assays, with manual or automated analytical procedures. Each point
represents the mean value of assays carried out in at least ten
laboratories using the same procedure, usually from more than one
continent and often from all five continents. There is a method-
dependent, reproducible difference between mean values.

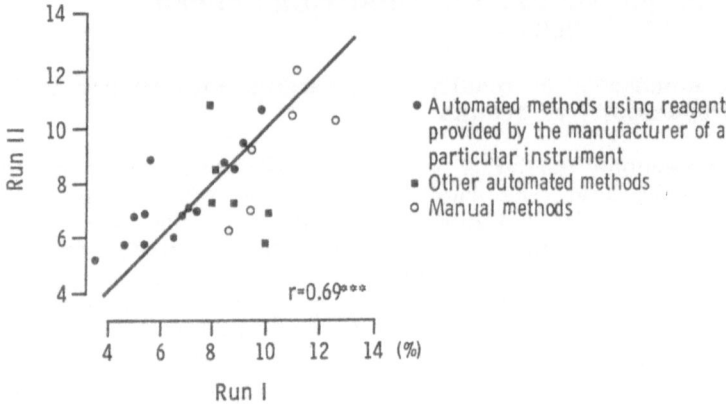

Figure 18.3   Serum bilirubin; correlation between method variance (CV)

Figure 18.3 shows the within-method precision for the same manual and automated methods. The overall precision for a particular analytical procedure is fairly predictable. Automated methods have better precision than manual ones. Automated methods with reagents provided by the manufacturer of a particular instrument tend to show less variability of long-term precision than automated methods where different types of reagents are used. The conclusions that can be drawn from Figure 18.3 are that:

-       The quality of this assay in terms of accuracy and precision is mainly determined by the combination of kit and instrument, and to a much lesser extent by local skills;

-       There still is quite a wide variation between procedures with regard to imprecision;

-       The situation (as illustrated in both Figures) has most likely not changed considerably over the last decade; and

-       The situation could reflect a certain degree of reluctance by industry to improve its products because of a lack of improved quality specification requirements forthcoming from the professional societies.

Obviously the problem is worthy of a tripartite discussion as would occur in ECCLS. Such discussions would involve all branches of the clinical laboratory sciences, resulting in a reasonably general solution that should be based on sound theoretical principles and appropriately adjusted to financial and technical realities.

The continued development of standards to maintain quality of work in the clinical laboratory sciences

An impressive range of European committee work already going on in this field takes advantage of the integrated approach ECCLS can offer, where science, health policies and industrial skills can blend to find optimal solutions.

One area of particular importance is the development of investigations for direct use by people themselves, whether ill or not, at home or outside the direct supervision of physicians and clinical laboratory scientists. This development could have considerable potential for maintaining and improving health, if implemented correctly from medical, economic and industrial points of view. It seems that ECCLS is ideally placed to support this effort on a voluntary basis by producing necessary guidelines that can be updated periodically to suit changing demands.

CONCLUSIONS

The outcome of these activities would certainly help to maintain and improve health in the future, as is illustrated in a simple way in Figure 18.4.

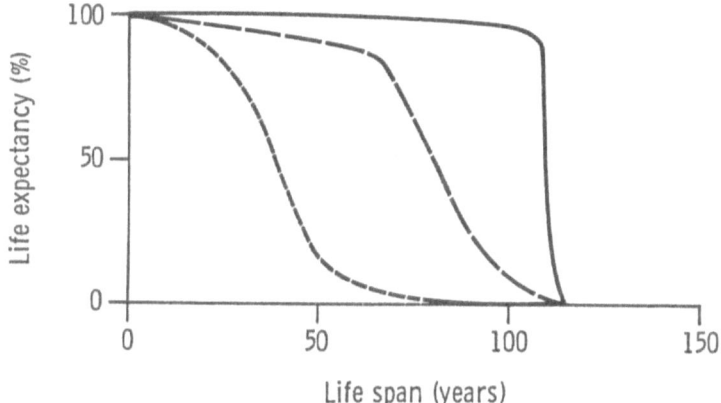

Figure 18.4 Life expectancy vs. life span during the early 20th century (– – – –), today (— — —) and in the optimum situation (———)

In the graph, life expectancy is plotted against life span for three different times: the early 20th century, today and the optimal situation. There is no evidence that life span has increased during the last century, and our maximal life span can be considered a biological constant that might be attainable if the 'machinery' is well maintained from a biological point of view. This constant is about 115 years according to The Guinness Book of Records. Could we maintain everybody to his or her 115th birthday? Life expectancy is increasing, but pushing life expectancy up to its maximum will require a lot more standardized knowledge about non-health. ECCLS can contribute to this push, helping to implement the goals of WHO for health in Europe in the year 2000.